CHIROPRA(

Greetings"

nay the years ahead be filled, with

Health Hope and Happiness"
for you and yours .

Arthur J Scofield D.O. F.rab.

"CHIROPRACTICE"
REVISED EDITION 1981
£3-75p

CHIROPRACTICE

The Science of Specific Spinal Adjustment

by
ARTHUR G. SCOFIELD, D.C., F.P.A.C.
(Fellow, The Palmer Academy of Chiropractic)

THORSONS PUBLISHERS LIMITED
Wellingborough, Northamptonshire

First published 1968
Second Impression 1973
Third Impression 1977
Second Edition (revised) 1981

To my wife, Nada Lilian
for her loyalty, help and devotion

© ARTHUR G. SCOFIELD 1968, 1981

British Library Cataloguing in Publication Data

Scofield, Arthur G.
  Chiropractice,
  1. Osteopathy
  I. Title
  615'5'33   RZ341

  ISBN 0-7225-0702-X

Printed in England by Nene Litho, Earls Barton, Northants.
Bound by Weatherby Woolnough, Wellingborough, Northants.

Contents

List of Illustrations

Preface

The purpose of this book is to enlighten those not already acquainted with Chiropractice, the largest *natural* healing profession in the world today, how it was re-discovered, by whom, and why it is so successful in the restoration to health of many who failed to respond to the efforts made on their behalf by their conscientious family physician. The physician is often at a loss when dealing with disease and disability frequently caused by spinal misalignments and vertebral subluxations; these in turn are followed by an inflammation of the nerve roots that tend to interfere with the function of the nerves which they supply.

While there are conditions in man that make it impossible for chiropractice, any more than the other healing arts, to be a sure cure for *all* diseases, nevertheless its application produces a remarkably high percentage of recoveries from disability and disease when all else has failed.

In this day and age, with so many new discoveries by the surgeon, medical doctor, scientist and engineer, it is quite easy to re-discover something for which credit rightly belongs to some person or group of the past.

Many writings and papers submitted by orthodox and unorthodox branches of the healing professions tend to create, by accident or design, the impression that spinal subluxations and misalignments are a contributory cause of some diseases, and their correction by spinal manipulations are worthy of acclaim as *new discoveries*. This is in spite of the fact that a Canadian, Daniel David Palmer, re-discovered the science in 1895, and his son, Bartlett Joshua Palmer, D.C., Ph.C., spent over fifty years of his life on its development and research, to give its results to the world through his lectures and writings while President of the first Chiropractic College 1906–1961.

Chiropractice presents a somewhat different approach to the healing arts from medicine, therefore some new words and interpretations are used and are listed under a "glossary of Chiropractic terminology".

As the science was re-discovered and developed by the Palmers it is inevitable that references to their talks, quotations, and writings will frequently appear in this book. Naturally, modern presentation of chiropractice will at times differ from some of the principles and practices taught by the developer, B. J. Palmer, and while quoting them as a review, it does not necessarily mean that they are entirely acceptable to the present-day Doctor of Chiropractice.

On certain points all are agreed that the science and art of chiropractice deals with the relationships between the articulations of the spinal column and the nervous system, and the role of these relationships in the restoration and maintenance of health.

While the chiropractic concept has been mentioned by various philosophers and doctors throughout the ages, the development of effective skills for the successful correction of spinal misalignments and other skeletal structures of the body is a relatively recent advance.

Since the human spine is particularly prone to misalignments and subluxations which, in turn, disrupt other bodily processes, thereby causing interference with their function, there is an increasing need for skilled doctors in science, who are prepared to devote their lives to this branch of the healing profession.

Every day, throughout the world, doctors of chiropractice utilize their professional education and special skills in a battle for the health of mankind.

Specially trained in the science and art of chiropractice these doctors regularly meet the ever-present challenge of a wide range of disorders, malfunctions and injuries that directly or indirectly can be attributed to spinal and other malpositions of the skeletal structures in man.

An attempt has been made to devote the earlier chapters of this book to the layman (particularly those who as yet have little knowledge of the science) and the latter to the legal and medical professions, and students. Where this has failed, it is because a separation would deprive a chapter of the information which should be common knowledge to both layman and professional.

Chiropractice – Present Role and Future Function

In medical terms, chiropractice is an entirely manipulative art, based on understanding of the spinal column and nervous system and their role in maintaining normal health, without the use of drugs or surgery.

In practice, the science consists of analysis of any interference with normal transmission of nerve energy from brain through Occipital Foramen, spinal column and other osseus tissue, principally through subluxations of spinal vertebrae, with subsequent compression of spinal cord or its ramifications through the intervertebral foramina. Any form of interference may be revealed by physical examination, radiography, neurocalograph or other sensitive instruments designed to measure nerve impulses.

Correction of abnormal deviation of the vertebral column's bony articulations is achieved by manual adjustment after careful study of the patient's spinograph.

Chiropractice was known to the ancient Greeks, Egyptians, Chinese and Hindus over 32 centuries ago but, when medical science discarded its Hippocratic principles in favour of chemical healing, chiropractice was neglected and ultimately forgotten.

Revival of interest in the subject did not occur till the 1890's when a Canadian 'Magnetic Healer', Daniel David Palmer, took an interest in the much discussed 'Osteopathic School' founded by Dr. Still and his associates in 1895. Palmer became particularly interested in their method of treatment of dislocations, subluxations and manipulation of cartilage.

After extensive study, Palmer became convinced that spinal subluxations were the basic cause of many of man's bodily diseases. He considered that the weakness of one or more bodily organs or tissues was caused by interference with the nervous system and its distribution, particularly at the source of emission from the spinal cord, i.e., the intervertebral foramina.

Palmer, born at Port Perry, Ontario, Canada, employed a janitor called Harvey Lillard who had lost his hearing many years previously. Lillard was persuaded to become the subject of an experiment when examination of his spinal column revealed a vertebra in an apparently abnormal position. Following palpation, Palmer gave the offending vertebra a manual thrust and, to the shock and surprise of both men, Lillard's hearing was promptly restored.

I, personally, confirmed this account in an interview with Lillard's grand-daughter during a visit by her to the Palmer College of Chiropractice, at Davenport, Iowa, U.S.A. The interview took place during one of my annual visits to the college which I regard as my 'alma mater'.

It was a wonderful coincidence that X-rays were discovered in the same year that Palmer made his own discovery. Chiropractice could now incorporate radiology into the field of spinal correction returning the art of spinal manipulation to the profession of healing.

Daniel David Palmer (born 1845, died 1913) named and recreated the Science of Chiropractice in 1895 and, in a primitive way, instructed several men on the effectiveness of spinal adjustments in the control and cure of ailments which showed symptoms of spinal distortion. For his trouble he was arrested and convicted of practising medicine – yes, medicine – without a licence because in those days no clear-cut distinction was made between orthodox medicine and the new science.

Palmer's son, Bartlett Joshua Palmer was born in 1881 and died in 1961. He became the recognised developer of the Art and Science of Chiropractice. 'B.J.', as he became widely known, was one of the select few to receive instruction from his father. Other notable names of the period included T.F. Haldledge, John A. Howard, Alva A. Gregory, Wellard Carver, S.M. Langworthy and Joy Loban. There were others but these are the names I remember best as mentioned by B.J. during our studies in the mid-twenties at what was then known as the Palmer School of Chiropractic. The school was started about 1905 by members of the group just mentioned, with B.J. Palmer as the principal driving force – a characteristic for which he was notable.

Daniel David Palmer, the founder, left Iowa about 1906, as did another two of the original group, to start other Chiropractic schools, such as the Universal and the National.

Palmer's grandson, the son of B.J., known as David D. Palmer, was born on 12th January 1906. He graduated from the University of Pennsylvania, became president of the Palmer College and was chiefly responsible for upgrading the original School to its present high status as a College.

I find no better answer to the question of 'What is chiropractice?' than to quote an excerpt from an article which appeared three years ago in the Journal of the Edinburgh Medical School, entitled 'Synapse', written by that fine expressive writer, Malcolm Kerr. He wrote: 'Perhaps one of the oddest situations of imbalance of status in public opinion with respect to clinical skills and effectiveness is that of the profession of Chiropractice. In terms of training the licensed chiropractor has learned skills which are comparable to, though different from, those of doctors and dentists.

His five-year training course has a similar content and extent to our own medical courses. The chiropractic profession has its own demanding ethical standards. Yet the law in this country offers no statutory protection whatsoever to the profession against the improper use of the term "Chiropractor". It is our responsibility as health students to understand the contradictions of this situation and, possibly, to rectify them.'

What then is chiropractice? Is it simply manipulation? Does it concern itself only with maladies of the spinal cord?

The prospectus from a major American College of Chiropractice explains: 'A Doctor of Chiropractice is a physician concerned with the health needs of the public as a member of the healing arts. He gives particular attention to the relationship of the structural and neurological aspects of the body in health and disease.

The prospectus continues to point out that the purpose of a chiropractor's professional education is to prepare him as a doctor to diagnose, including spinal analysis, and care for the human body in health and disease, and consult or refer to other physicians.

The chiropractic profession is dedicated to providing the public with thorough and complete drugless health care.

Doctors of Chiropractice, as primary physicians, are one of the three major portals of entry into the U.S. health care delivery system.

Chiropractic therapeutics utilize adjustive and manipulative procedures and other drugless procedures, physiological therapeutics, dietary correction and supplementation, kinesiology and rehabilitative procedures, to aid in restoration of anatomical relationships and physiological capabilities.

Malcolm Kerr points out that chiropractice is a young science but its progress in the Twentieth Century has been rapid, particularly in those areas of healing which have been neglected by orthodox medicine.

The profession is well-established in the Americas where there are 13 colleges, each with between 500 and 2,000 students and has fairly recently opened an Anglo-European College of Chiropractice in Bournemouth, England.

Mr. Kerr suggests that, in general, there is very little antagonism between chiropractors and neurologists, rheumatologists and radiologists, who recognise the fine contribution which chiropractors have made to research in their fields, for example, in the development of Cine-X-radiography.

Mr. Kerr adds: 'Any doubt about the nature or thoroughness of chiropractic training is dispelled by reference to a Chiropractic College prospectus. The academic requirements are taxing and college regulations appear to be more strict than would be tolerated by students here. The degree awarded after five years successful completion of the course is Doctor of Chiropractic (D.C.) which confers the same conventional courtesy title of Doctor as does a medical first degree'.

'The profession's ethical standards are laid down by the British Chiropractors' Association, the official body, and more or less the profession's equivalent of the British Medical Association.

'It is an unfortunate side-effect of the National Health Service and provision of health care, regardless of the patient's means, that bureaucracy and domination of the N.H.S. by the medical profession has excluded the valuable services offered by Doctors of Chiropractice and other healers.

'It has deprived many patients, sentenced by orthodox medicine to prolonged pain or illness, of access to the skills needed for the restoration of their problems which can only be remedied by Government support for Chiropractic Colleges and official recognition of the profession's contributions to health care.'

From time to time the question of acceptance of chiropractice and osteopathy into the National Health Service is debated. During one such debate in the House of Lords in 1974, the suggestion was made that chiropractice could be taken on as an 'auxilliary' to the medical profession.

Later, this point was discussed by many of the Doctors of Chiropractice who agreed that they could never submit to becoming auxiliaries to medical doctors who had not achieved the training or experience in the science of chiropractice to attain the same high professional skills in specific spinal adjustments.

Legal recognition, it was agreed, would do much to eliminate the unscrupulous persons who presented themselves as chiropractors, after taking crash courses of seven to ten days, and who then engaged in blatant advertising. Similar legal recognition could be extended to osteopaths and naturopaths but, as far as chiropractice was concerned, its practitioners would only welcome this type of recognition if their science was accepted as an independent profession in the healing world.

The U.S.A. has already given a lead. In October, 1972, Congress voted to include chiropractic services within the Medicare Programme on a limited but permanent basis. In addition, Congress adopted a provision on health maintenance organisations or comprehensive group health service organisations which required that chiropractice must be included in their programmes before they could receive Federal funds as Medicare providers.

It has been estimated that the number of patients utilising chiropractic professional services in Canada, the U.S.A. and Mexico totals over 30 million. The work has to be spread between some 20,000 Doctors of Chiropractice.

Today chiropractic doctors are often asked to lecture at medical schools in the U.S.A. They enjoy recognition in every State and Province of the U.S.A. and Canada.

With the acceptance of the recommended two years' pre-chiropractic college requirements and the eventual recognition of an official accrediting agency by the Department of Health, Education and Welfare (U.S.A.) in 1974, combined with the Government grant for the University of Colorado Chiropractic Research Project, under the direction of Chung-Ha Suh, Ph.D. and Martin Luttges, Ph.D., there is a large intake of qualified students in the 13 chiropractic colleges of the U.S.A., Canada and the Anglo-European College.

Graduations from the colleges exceed 1,000 a year. In Gt. Britain there are just over 100 Doctors of Chiropractice registered with the B.C.A. and about 75 Associate Members, of whom over 40 are British, in the Anglo-European College.

Taken from an article by the author which appeared in the Journal of the Research Society of Natural Therapeutics.

The Scofield Biography

Many of the British pioneers who went out to Canada during the Victorian era exemplified the spirit of independence and sturdy individualism born of an age which set little store by social welfare benefits.

They were the men who carved farmsteads out of the virgin bush, founded new industries, discovered mineral wealth, and built up the country to the point where it could afford to export a few pioneers – newspaper magnates, and industrialists, who returned to the land of their forbears to introduce new ways of thinking, a fresh approach to life.

People like Lord Beaverbrook and Lord Thomson may have made the headlines in more respects than one, but Canadian born Dr. Arthur Scofield remains a pioneer who, in one slight but wiry figure, combines the attributes of a Victorian pioneer with the fervour of an old-time evangelist in his continued fight for the acceptance of Chiropractice in Britain.

The one remaining major ambition in the life of the man who is already accepted as "the father of British Chiropractice" is to see that treatment becomes available to all through the National Health Service. When this day arrives it will complete the full cycle of a life which has spanned the best part of a revolutionary century, and yet managed to combined the best characteristics of two contrasting ages.

"Doc", as he is affectionately known to colleagues and patients alike, continues to work full-time in his Suffolk Clinic, though he long since passed the age when lesser men would have retired to tend their roses.

The "Doc" is a small man, slightly stooped, with a shock of fair hair which stands up on end. He speaks with a modulated boom of a voice, which still betrays his Canadian origins although he has lived in England since 1932. His eyes burn with the intensity of a prophet, and his enthusiasm for his vocation remains undiminished. He will not be talking long before he reveals fresh ideas and new plans to help sufferers from back-trouble and allied ailments.

Some indication of his way of thinking may be gleaned from his invariable use of the expression "Dis-ease", which indicates an approach very different from the orthodox. Another aspect of the character of the man is revealed in the fact that he once was a physical "write-off", an 80 per cent. cripple as a teenager, who much later in his career, was forced to retire prematurely because of blindness, which, fortunately, proved to be temporary.

When he was 16 years old Arthur Scofield lied about his age, giving the authorities to understand that he was 18, and old enough to join the Canadian 37th Infantry Battalion. He saw action on the Somme till the day when he was buried alive by an explosive shell. Completely buried by tons of earth, only Scofield's hands showed above the ground. They were seen by a comrade who brought a rescue party to dig him out.

During succeeding months Scofield was seen by British and Canadian Army doctors and by specialists. There was nothing that they could do for the young man who was apparently destined for the vegetable existence of a helpless cripple. Then one day, a chance meeting was to alter the whole course of Scofield's life.

Into the Winnipeg General Hospital came Dr. Frank McElrea, a chiropractor, who volunteered to take the patient back to his own home. Slowly, methodically, Dr. McElrea worked on the young soldier's spine, gradually adjusting it back into position, till eventually he was fully restored to health.

In those days Chiropractice was still in its infancy, regarded with the suspicion that orthodox medicine always reserves for the "fringe sciences". It had been Arthur Scofield's intention to qualify as a medical doctor, but, following his "miracle" recovery, he decided to enrol in the Palmer College of Chiropractice in the mid-West State of Iowa and qualify as a "Doctor of Chiropractice".

On graduation he set out to build up his own private practice in Canada. When his father, who was living in the Channel Isles, became ill during 1932, Dr. Scofield came over to nurse him during the final months of his life.

During this period he moved to Bury St Edmunds in Suffolk where one night "Doc" attended a party given by a prominent local businessman, whose daughter was a complete cripple following an accident when she was a 12 month-old baby. The little girl had been dropped accidentally and was incapable of walking or talking.

Dr. Scofield volunteered to treat the girl. Within six weeks she began to talk, and within three months was capable of walking.

As a result of the girl's recovery the news soon spread, and before long, Dr. Scofield received so many inquiries from prospective patients that he had to give up the idea of returning home to Canada, and he set up practice in Bury St Edmunds. Later, because of the number of patients who travelled down from London to attend the Clinic, Dr. Scofield decided it would be more convenient for them if he moved to Ingrams Well, Sudbury.

The practice flourished till the outbreak of War when petrol rationing was introduced. Immediately following Chamberlain's message of "Peace in our time", the instincts of an old soldier inspired Dr Scofield to build the first "dug-out" air raid shelter in Sudbury, and to join the Home Guard. He was made Sudbury Town Military Commander, with full responsibility for all emergency services.

When the War came to an end "Doc" resumed his practice. When he had first arrived in England he was one of only ten Chiropractors in the country, and the only one with a practice in East Anglia. At the end of the War there were still very few working, but their value was becoming increasingly recognized.

Dr. Scofield was kept fully stretched. As Chiropractors will not work on a patient without first taking x-ray pictures of the spinal column, "Doc" was constantly exposed to the effects of secondary radiation, in the form of x-ray dermatitis which affected his hands, feet, and eventually, his eyes.

He could no longer continue his work. He left his practice promising to return when fit enough, and moved to the Highlands of Scotland for a complete rest over the next two years. The fresh air and constant walking, with the long-range views, began to restore his sight, and the moment that he had recovered his health, he returned to his adopted home at Sudbury to set up practice in the present Clinic.

The practice steadily built up to the point where the Clinic now deals with over 200 patients in a week, over half of them treated personally by the "Doc", who has always been concerned that the benefits of the science should not simply be confined to those who could afford the fees.

As a result, he was instrumental in setting up the Scofield Chiropractice Charity Trust with the backing of prominent businessmen and women – one provided an individual donation of £10,000 – and other volunteers. Believed to be the first Chiropractic Charity Trust to be set up in any country (the Trust was formed in 1964) to enable people of limited means to avail themselves of treatment.

The Trustees have raised an average of £1,000 a year through such activities as fêtes and raffles, and patients can receive a free course of treatment; and, if necessary, transport can also be provided. As their contribution to the Trust the Doctors cut their fees by one third.

The Trust also administers scholarships to students of Chiropractice, including pupils at the only British College in Bournemouth. These scholarships are only awarded on merit to deserving cases. A condition is that after graduation the student must practice in Great Britain for a period of at least two years.

At present there are still only about a hundred Doctors of Chiropractice working in Britain. By the end of the decade Dr. Scofield hopes that the figure will be closer to a thousand, when there will be sufficient qualified men and women to serve every major centre of population in the country.

When this point is reached and every citizen can avail himself of chiropractic health care, Dr. Scofield has been assured that the National Health Service will accept responsibility so that nobody in need of treatment will be denied it because of expense. The old pioneer is confident that he will see the culmination of his lifetime's work in the full acceptance of the science by the authorities – providing that he lives as long as his grandmother did, and she reached the age of 91.

Dr. Scofield has every reason to be optimistic for, apart from his own experience under British conditions, he has seen the advance of Chiropractice in the United States and Canada, which generally set the trends which Britain follows ten years later. At one stage Chiropractice was outlawed in some States, and the doctor was liable to imprisonment for practising his profession!

In October 1972 the Congress of the United States voted to include chiropractic services within the Medicare programme on a limited but permanent basis. In addition, Congress adopted a provision on "health maintenance organizations" or comprehensive group health service organizations which required that Chiropractice must be included in their programmes before they could receive Federal funds as Medicare providers.

As part of the enabling legislation the definition of "physician" was extended to cover a licensed Chiropractor whose qualifications conformed to uniformed minimum standards.

His services would be covered under the programme as "physicians' services" but only with respect to treatment of the spine by means of manual manipulation which the Chiropractor is legally authorised to perform. Claims for such treatment would have to be verifiable with a satisfactory x-ray indicating the existence of a subluxation of the spine.

On Tuesday, 18 December 1973, President Nixon signed the Health, Education and Welfare and Labour Department Appropriation Bill, and for the first time two million dollars were earmarked for Chiropractic Research under the National Institute of Neurological Disease and Stroke of the National Institute of Health.

To help in establishing a similar wider acceptance and understanding of the role of the science in Britain, Dr. Scofield has been instrumental in forming the British Pro-Chiropractic Association.

In 1966 Dr. Scofield was the first European-based Doctor to be elected a Fellow of the Palmer College of Chiropractice, the "fountainhead" of the science, to which he has returned annually for research seminars and to keep abreast of current developments.

He has been separately honoured as a 50-year graduate of the College, and more recently Dr. Scofield was awarded a fellowship in the Research Society of Natural Therapeutics in England.

Rintoul Booth
Aldham, Suffolk

Rintoul Booth

Rintoul Booth, edited the first edition of *Chiropractice* in 1968, when he was still an agricultural editor and broadcaster.

Shortly afterwards he abandoned this career to become a full-time sculptor of animals in bronze and steel, following exhibitions in London and elsewhere. But, sadly, he died in 1979 aged 46.

His work is to be found in private collections all over the world, and his major public work is a life-size Black Bull, of welded steel strip, situated at the entrance of The East Suffolk Institute of Agriculture at Otley, West Yorkshire.

The idea of a "Universal Intelligence" which, he said, he discovered from my original manuscript, was central to Rintoul Booth's development of a unique system of engineering of animal forms in sculpture.

Rintoul Booth was listed in the 1976 edition of the International Authors and Writers, *Who's Who*, as the author of a number of books on farming and equestrian subjects varying in approach, from the factual to the satirical. He shared with the author the honour of appearing in the International edition of *Men of Achievement*.

Arthur G. Scofield, F.P.A.C., F.R.S.N.T.

Introduction

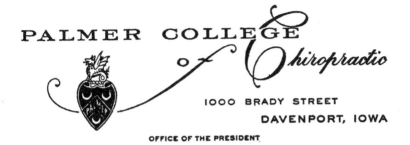

PALMER COLLEGE of Chiropractic

1000 BRADY STREET
DAVENPORT, IOWA

OFFICE OF THE PRESIDENT

June 1966

The story of chiropractic, its discovery, its development and its evolution as an art, science and philosophy, since its discovery by my grandfather, Daniel David Palmer, September 18, 1895, to its present position as the leading drugless healing art, is a very interesting subject.

The chiropractic patient of today, as well as the average lay person, has little understanding of the processes of evolution through which chiropractic has gone in its 70 years. The purpose of this book is to acquaint the reader with the many steps through which it has gone to reach its present recognized scientific position in the healing arts.

Dr. Arthur G. Scofield, D.C., M.B.C.A., the author of this book, is well known to me. He is eminently qualified to write on this subject, having been for many years a student and practitioner of the chiropractic philosophy, science and art, as well as closely identified in person and spirit with the Palmer family and the fountainhead of the profession . . . the Palmer College of Chiropractic, Davenport, Iowa, U.S.A.

I have had the good fortune of knowing Dr. Arthur Scofield personally for many years and it's a relationship that I cherish.

I am sure this presentation will be most interesting. It will add greatly to the appreciation and respect of the chiropractic health service.

(Signed) DAVID D. PALMER
President

CHAPTER ONE

An Explanation and a History

To most people chiropractice is a little known and somewhat mysterious word. They may have heard of it distantly, or know people who have been to see a chiropractor for their "slipped disc". As chiropractice is not yet an officially recognized branch of healing in Britain, a patient usually only hears of its benefit to health through friends, as the literature on the subject is scanty.

Many of my patients who have been apparently cured of complaints such as the incorrectly named "slipped disc", within a comparatively short time, consider the recovery of health as miraculous, and wish to know more about the science. But no science can be formulated without an art and philosophy.

The purpose of this book is to explain these principles for the benefit of the interested layman and in its later chapters explain in greater detail to the potential student, or doctor of medicine, who is prepared to approach the subject with an open mind.

Chiropractice as a word sounds complicated, but is derived from two Greek words Cheir and Praktos. Cheir is the word surgeon, in its older form Chirurgeon, and Praktos means hand, which in turn gives us such words as practically, practical, and practice. Linked together, the two words simply mean "done by hand"; done skilfully.

In fact, chiropractice remains an entirely manipulative art based on an understanding of the spinal column and nervous system and its role in maintaining normal health, without the use of drugs or surgery.

The chiropractor believes that much disease, the meaning of which becomes clearer if written "dis-ease", or to use another expression, abnormal function, is caused by interference with nerve transmission and expression, due to pressure, strain or tension upon the spinal cord or spinal nerves, as a result of bony segments of the vertebral column deviating from their normal position.

The practise of chiropractice consists of analysis of any interference with normal nerve transmission and expression. This analysis may be carried out by making use of x-ray equipment and other sensitive instruments designed to measure nerve impulses. Correction is undertaken by manual adjustment of the abnormal deviation of the bony articulations of the vertebral column. Thus normal nerve transmission is restored to maintain health.

It must be emphasized from the outset that no use is made either of drugs or surgery. At a time when the question of drug taking is featured in every popular newspaper in the country, it cannot be over-emphasized that the taking of any type of drug will interfere with the balance of the normal nervous system and make it impossible to undertake corrective manipulation to achieve restoration of normal health.

To clear up another popular misconception, chiropractice is not a branch of osteopathy. An osteopath will undertake to treat a patient without first taking an x-ray of the spinal column. A patient, coming to a chiropractor, cannot expect to be treated immediately. He must first be x-rayed. The chiropractor will closely study the pictures, primarily only to find out the extent of the deviations of the spinal articulations. Equally important, he will carry out a close examination to discover any fractures or fundamental weaknesses. In these cases the chiropractor will recommend that the patient should see his doctor of medicine, or a specialist. Chiropractice does not claim to be a cure-all but a complementary branch of medical science. Where it does cure an apparent disorder, such as lumbago or sciatica, it merely restores previously interrupted nerve function to normal.

Another fallacy appears to be that the doctor of chiropractice, in some way, is not as well qualified as his colleague in medicine. In a later chapter the reader may compare similar medical and chiropractic courses offered in the United States and Canada where chiropractice is officially recognized. I look forward to the day when this will be the case in Britain. At the moment there is still a degree of prejudice in certain quarters; the same type of prejudice which led many American States to pass laws forbidding chiropractors to carry out their science on pain of imprisonment. Fortunately, this prejudice has never reached such lengths in Britain, and each year, as knowledge grows, there is developing a better understanding and acceptance of the profession. If this book serves to increase this understanding it will have fully served its purpose.

In this age of scepticism the idea of God or a Universal Intelligence is frequently discounted by scientists and it would seem by certain Bishops. These people are entitled to their views but the chiropractor must base his art and practice on the philosophy that a Universal Source of Intelligence does exist. Within every human being there is a part of this Greater Intelligence which D. D. Palmer, the Canadian who re-discovered the science in 1895, described as "Innate Intelligence". He differentiated between the three sources of bodily control as Universal Intelligence, meaning the Outer Force or Power. This is continued as "Innate Intelligence" which directs every function of the body every second of the day, throughout life. Part of the Innate Intelligence can be adapted for conscious use within the body by means of education, to give educated intelligence.

Whether or not one wishes to accept the idea of a Universal Source of Intelligence, nobody has yet been able to define precisely how the Innate Intelligence draws a blueprint of every organ of the body, builds, organizes and assembles each of them, then starts and keeps them running. The scientists have started to discover some of these secrets, and each year brings another part of the answer to fit in to the complete jigsaw, While all this is going on this Innate or Internal Natural Intelligence continues to know when to make you sneeze, blow your nose, blink your eyes, how to heal a cut, or mend a fractured bone, raise a blister when the skin is burned, grow hair and nails. This intelligence tells you when you are thirsty, hungry or sleepy. It directs, regulates, governs and controls all functions in all bodies all the time. Innate Intelligence knows when something is wrong, where, how much, what needs rebuilding, and how to do it. It is this same intelligence, force, or call it what you will, which has the power to make any sick organ well.

As long as this Innate Intelligence within you controls your body a state of "health" exists. Should something interfere with normal control of that internal power, a state of "dis-ease" arises.

Science has taught us to recognize when disease in specific areas are appropriately named. You can be suffering specifically from cardiac disease, kidney disease, or more precisely from valvular heart disease, ulcerated stomach disease, nephritis, describing a kind of kidney disease, but whatever name is given, is a failure of the Innate Intelligence properly to regulate body function.

The chiropractor maintains that Innate Intelligence controls all body functions through the nervous system. If some factor causes a disturbance in the nerves that would interfere with thought transmission from the brain, then at the end of the nerve you begin to feel a state of dis-ease whether in organ, tissue, and/or periphery.

Chiropractice is a method used to release interference to nerve supply so that the "power within" can heal you. The doctor of chiropractice is equipped with instruments which tell him when trouble has developed in the nerves. He then does everything possible to help this Innate Intelligence to heal your body by removing obstructions which are causing interference with the distribution of nerve impulses. The doctor is not "healing" you because this power is above and beyond the control of any man. All he can do to produce healing for you is make the correct adjustment to restore the full innate power.

There is nothing new in this science which was known to the Greeks, the Ancient Egyptians, Chinese and Hindus, more than thirty-two centuries ago. Hippocrates, who is acknowledged by many to be the Father of Healing and the Inspiration behind the well-known "Hippocratic Oath" which governs the professional conduct of the physicians, stated "look well to the spine for the cause of disease". Hippocrates evidently understood the importance of the spinal column to health maintenance, a fact which has frequently been neglected. Medical science branched off on its own path, chiropractice was neglected and fell into dis-use until Palmer accidentally re-discovered it. He spent the rest of his life in developing the theory which has now given rise to the modern practice.

Ancient manuscripts and other documents contain concise but clear descriptions of chiropractice. Amongst the most ancient is an Egyptian papyrus which dates probably to the seventeenth century before Christ. Translated by the late Professor James Henry Breasted, the Egyptian papyrus is now known as the Edwin Smith or Papyrus of New York, which under File R.A.C.1291dd British Library was published and translated by the Oriental Institute of Chicago University (1930) in two original volumes.

In it the following chiropractic cases treated by spinal adjustment are described:

> Sprain of cervical vertebrae.
> Dislocation of cervical vertebrae.
> Displacement of cervical vertebrae.
> Crushed cervical vertebrae.
> Sprain in a spinal vertebra.

It was not only the ancient Hindus, Chinese, Babylonians, Assyrians, Egyptians, the aboriginals of Ceylon and the Brazilians of the Matto Grosso, but the highly specialized Incas and Aztecs and other American Indians who used their hands for curative purposes.

Practised manipulation in some form or other has been employed by all mankind. The systematic and intelligent teaching of chiropraxy, as it was originally known was undertaken by the Priests of the mythical semi-gods and heroes of Greece. Two of the most important teachers were the Thessalians, Aesculapius and Chiron, The Centaur, who were the first instructors in the arts of Grecian classical medicine. Through them, and their descendants, the different therapeutic methods have been transmitted to all civilized mankind. Various bas-reliefs left by the Greeks bear mute witness to applied rachiotherapy, surgery, and other medical branches. Aesculapius long ago called the attention of the practitioner to the fact that if the various spinal deformities or the different vertebral displacements, large or small, are not properly corrected in time, serious complications are likely to result, to the deterioration of individual health.

In the Sydenham Society's edition of "The Genuine works of Hippocrates" there is the following translation of his observations on the subject of the spine: "One or more spinal vertebrae go out of place, not very much from the rest, but just slightly one gives way from the other. These vertabrae, one or more, do not have to get out of their place very much in order to produce discomfort to the patient, but if one or more do go out of place very much, this may cause death."

For many centuries the Chinese employed the method of rubbing the bones of the neck. They applied pressure with a copper coin in this region to ease ailments of the nerves. Rock carvings made centuries ago in Egypt show healers placing their hands along the spinal nerve column. The wonderful endurance of the North American Indians is attributed to the care given by the squaw mother who binds the little "papoose" child to a board until its spine assumes the primary curves essential to proper development. In another part of the world, the Maoris of New Zealand still practise the ancient habit of walking bare-foot on the spine of a prone person to cure certain ailments.

In an article by Roger Davenport appears the following description: "From one of the smallest booths peals of laughter rang out in unbroken succession. A naked woman was lying on her stomach over a bench and, on her back, a pretty little girl of seven or eight was performing a most ferocious war-dance jumping and kicking with her little feet on the living platform. Both were in fits of laughter and seemed to be equally amused by their queer occupation. Questioned as to its object the woman replied, between bursts of laughter, that her digestion had gone wrong and nothing was so good for it as this was, it was already much better and would soon be all right if only the youngster could keep it up long enough. This apparently strange healing custom was reported by Prince William of Sweden when on a visit to Rangoon."

History records a blacking out of early scientific findings during the Dark Ages, until in the early seventeenth century, chiropractice was re-discovered by the great French philosopher, Descartes, who emphasized the importance of the nervous system working through body muscles as a major influence in its reaction to environment. The re-discovery was again allowed to lapse.

Not until 1895 did it make a reappearance. This time it was a Canadian, Dr. Daniel David Palmer (born Port Perry, Ontario, 7th March 1845), who discovered the principle on which modern chiropractice is based.

A janitor was employed in the building where Dr. Palmer had

his practice. The janitor, Harvey Lilliard, became deaf. Dr. Palmer adjusted the man's vertebrae in the neck and hearing was restored. From this discovery on 18th September 1895, made in a homely fashion by a simple adjustment of one vertebrae, begins the evolution of the entire science of chiropractice.

Dr. Palmer founded and became first President of a Chiropractic School (the Palmer Infirmary and Chiropractic Institute in Davenport, Iowa).

A rugged individualist, D. D. Palmer was an omnivorous reader of literature dealing with the previous experience and history of treating the sick. Believing that external agents in the treatment of disease were not the proper means of cure, he became interested in the natural phenomena of freeing the laws of nature from within man, thereby releasing the normal restorative (Innate Force of Universal Intelligence).

Because of this he became interested in the adjustment of subluxations (spinal displacements accompanied by nerve transmission interference), reasoning that if a correction of a spinal displacement in the neck producing restoration of hearing, then correction of other apparent spinal displacements should restore health to the organs and parts supplied by the particular nerves emanating from such vertebral malposition.

In simple language, by restoring the normal nerve force which he called "Innate or inborn intelligence", health would follow.

It was left to the mental endowment peculiar to the old master to re-discover the principle of chiropractice, since when millions of people have been given relief from sickness and disease as a result of Dr. Daniel David Palmer's genius and creative concept.

In August 1964 while attending a research seminar at the Palmer Chiropractic College I was privileged to meet the granddaughter of Harvey Lilliard (Dr. Palmer's first Chiropractic patient), who produced, by documentary evidence and conversation, proof of her grandfather's restoration of hearing through spinal adjustment.

There has been much opposition to chiropractice in the Medical World, but generally speaking, it is the leaders of organized medicine who fall into this group, not so much the rank and file, some even going so far as to refer to chiropractice as a "cult". Some have failed to examine it dispassionately, and therefore speak from prejudice or could it be ignorance? That this could well be the case is evident by one neurologist who stated that chiropractice does not seem reasonable as a theory and I believe there are no facts supporting the idea that disease may be caused by irritation or pressure on spinal nerve roots.

Some indication that professional prejudice exists was evident when the well-known orthopaedist John M. Mennell counselled doctors in the statement: "under certain circumstances I think you are justified in asking a well-trained manipulator, whoever he may be, to treat your patient for that specific complaint, just as you would ask a pharmacist to make up a prescription . . . Do not deprive your patients of relief from pain because of your prejudice".

Naturally, there is a philosophical difference between the viewpoints of orthodox medicine and chiropractice but time after time things happen in the world of research that bring both branches of healing into near parallel lines. For example, for many years, doctors of chiropractice held the view that the appendix in man should not be removed as a matter of routine. They considered it was not just a vestigial organ, but that it had a definite place and a definite part to play in the protection of the body. This was many years before its importance became generally known. An article expressing the latest medical opinion on this subject was published in the *Medical World News* in March 1966 to the effect that the appendix, far from being a vestigial organ, is a part of the body's immunological defence against certain kinds of cancer. The article suggested that appendices should not be removed as a routine procedure when operating on persons under thirty years of age for other complaints. Years ago, the Dean of a Chiropractic school rightly and wisely called in a medical doctor when his wife had a sudden attack of appendicitis. Upon his verification, it was decided to operate the following morning. But in the meantime, to ease the pain, the Dean treated his wife with cold compresses and a spinal adjustment. The pain and tenderness disappeared and the number of white corpuscles in the blood returned to normal. All agreed that the operation was no longer necessary, which seemed to underscore the basic difference in approach to health and disease. Chiropractors believe in the innate wisdom of the human organism and its inherent powers, and endeavour to assist it by removing obstruction to nerve distribution.

Sometimes however, more drastic measures are necessary, then drugs or surgery become vital.

But chiropractors believe in assisting the body to mend itself and, while chiropractice cannot do everything, what it can do, it does well. Therefore, where not contra-indicated, it is their belief that chiropractice should be tried before drugs or the knife.

There is an old French proverb which states "There are no diseases, only sick people", which is very much in accord with the opinion of chiropractors who prefer the term *dis-ease* (not at ease), rather than the medical term disease. In the 1920s the late noted physician Sir William Osler, when writing on Louis Pasteur's role in the progress of medicine in the nineteenth century, said: "We learned to trust Nature more and Drugs less. Much treatment was and still is irrational."

Probably one of the main reasons why the doctors of chiropractice succeed with so-called incurables is the appreciation and acknowledgement of the principle of body mechanics especially in relation to spinal balance, for it is absolutely essential that one part compensates for the malposition of any other part. The perfect example is the hunchback's spine which, having an abnormal posterior curve in the thoracic spine, is compensated by an abnormal anterior or forward tilt in the lumbar and pelvis. And, as the close relationship between the nervous system and the circulatory system can be considered of paramount importance to good health, any postural changes that affect the spinal vertebrae to the extent of producing compression of tissue surrounding nerve roots will upset this relationship to the extent of producing organ and tissue dis-ease.

The orthopaedists Maguson and Coulter stated, in 1920, that, "Unless the medical profession wakes up to the fact that our bodies are built upon mechanical principles and, that many things we have groped in the dark about are due to a mechanical fault . . . we are doing our patients a grave injustice, neglecting our duties as physicians." In *The Practitioner* of February 1934 one of England's leading orthopaedists, James Mennell, M.D., M.A., wrote: "It is indisputable that the testimony is overwhelming, that countless patients have derived relief from aches and pains of a great variety as a result of manipulation of the joints of the back. This is only what we should expect, once we realize that the joints in question are just as much joints in every detail as are those of the extremities. The only difference is that, from the very nature of their shape and movement and the stresses that are laid upon them, they are more liable to 'lock' with the creation of a 'lesion'. Local Pain would thus be caused, and relief would be reasonably expected to follow manipulative treatment if properly applied in suitable cases. It is thus that many patients claim, and quite rightly, the cure of widespread symptoms as the result of spinal manipulation."

There exists in Germany today an association of more than a thousand medical men with the name Medical Research and Action Society for Chiropractice, the purpose of which is to acquaint its members with the principles and mechanics of chiropractice, openly crediting chiropractice. G. Gutmann, M.D., of Hamm, Germany, writes: "On the basis of our experience accumulated over the years, we believe that we may declare that many treatments would be superfluous if the manipulative therapy called Chiropractic were applied to diagnosis, indications and technique." (Hippokrates, 15 th September 1957).

CHAPTER TWO

How it works, with reference to "Slipped Discs?", Lumbago and Sciatica

All body functions are co-ordinated and controlled by the nervous system, as many of the disabilities of mankind occur as the result of factors other than spinal displacements. Even though this involves the nervous system, it follows that such disabilities are not within the range of chiropractic. Should such cases come to the attention of the doctor of chiropractic, patients should and would be sent to their medical adviser.

On the other hand, patients who experience spinal misalignment problems that affect the neurological tissues of the spinal cord or its ramifications, may never recover completely, despite all the specialist's attention of the medical profession unless he receives corrective manipulations by a doctor of chiropractic.

A patient suffering from malfunction or a reduction of function in an organ can be relieved medically to a certain extent, but complete recovery is not possible if, at the same time, the nerves which supply the organ are adversely affected at the nerve root, or along its pathway from the spinal cord because of malposition or subluxation of one or more of the spinal vertebrae.

It is therefore to the advantage of all patients that a closer degree of co-operation should exist between medical doctors and chiropractic doctors. Better co-operation could result in a much higher standard of general health and give people a better understanding of their bodily functions.

As J. F. McAndrews, D.C., Ph.C., of the Palmer College faculty stated at the first national congress on chiropractice held in Chicago in 1967: "The public deserves an objective explanation of chiropractice. The brain, among other functions, is a cerebral mechanism which constantly and continually monitors the co-ordinated, integrated function of all of the body's anatomical structures or parts, by way of neurological or nerve pathways."

He described the spinal cord as an extension of the brain and, arising out of the spinal cord, as it passes downwards from the brain through the spinal column, are the spinal nerves. These nerves leave the spinal cord at somewhat regular intervals and, either directly provide communication between the brain and the part supplied, or do so, indirectly, by connecting up with other portions of the vast and complex network of nerves which govern the body's function.

Because of its high degree of vulnerability to a concussion of force, the spinal column, which houses the delicate spinal cord and the roots of the spinal nerves, may become distorted. One or more of the twenty-four movable segments of spine may become slightly to grossly misplaced, there may be a muscular fixture of one segment to another with no noticeable displacement or there may be a total dislocation.

In the event of the occurrence of a slight to gross misalignment, the chiropractor must locate and correct this or the chances for a malfunction of the nerve pathways involved is extremely great.

The chiropractic student must also be trained in the location of a spinal segment which no longer functions in the full range of its normal motion. This condition, in fact, only evidences itself upon a combination of highly specialized x-ray studies, observations, and motion examinations.

In the case of a total dislocation, the patient would be referred to a physician. Under ideal circumstances, the chiropractor would also present the results of his specialized findings to the physician so that the patient would receive the most knowledgeable care possible.

The exact nature of the alteration in the nerve impulse that occurs is not yet fully known but the extensive clinical and laboratory proof of the cause and effect relationship between a misplaced spinal segment resulting in neurological changes and a malfunctioning organ, has strongly established the relationship, and, of course, it is only a short time between malfunction and a resulting disease process.

Doctors of chiropractice realize the major role the spine and the nervous system play in controlling and maintaining normal functions of the organs and tissues of the body and with a comprehensive knowledge of human anatomy plus a carefully developed skill in application they manually correct malpositions of the body's bone structure particularly the vertebrae of the spine, and in order to maintain a healthy body, consistently endeavour to procure an accurate juxtaposition of the vertebral articulations.

The human spine is subjected to so many stresses and strains, through malpositions such as the occupational curvature developed in many cases by repetitive work on the assembly line, long periods of sitting in the modern low-slung car, the fixed intense gaze at the television, the whiplash effect of sudden car braking, the sudden shock to the golfer when he misses the putt and hits the divot, plus weakened back muscles because there is no time to walk any more.

So we find an ever increasing need for practitioners of the science of chiropractice to correct, among many other things, the old-fashioned cases of lumbago, and sciatica, which complaints have, over the years, developed into the much more fashionable so-called "slipped disc" or "herniated vertebral disc syndrome".

Science has proved that abnormal functioning and many disorders of the body are frequently caused by interference with nerve transmission, due to the pressure, strain, or tension placed upon the spinal cord, spinal nerve roots, and surrounding tissue, and in many cases a deviation from normal of the spinal vertebrae proved the key factor.

In the upper cervical spine, or neck region, we find misplaced vertebra producing a partial occlusion of the foramen magnum with subsequent compression surrounding the spinal cord, again there often exists a reduction of the intervertebral foramen (opening between the spinal vertebrae) due to malposition of vertebra and degeneration of the disc between, causing sufficient compression of the nerves emitting from this region to produce pain, numbness, and impaired function of the organs supplied by these nerves.

The task of your doctor of chiropractice, therefore, is to remove by spinal adjustments (applied by hand only) the bony pressure at the correct places where such occur.

These are discovered by physical examinations that reveal unnatural stance, limitations of movement, and restrictions in the placement of limbs.

Nerve inflammation is revealed by instrumentation such as the thermo-coupling detectors in instruments such as the neurocalometer and neurocalograph, which are placed at the point of exit of the nerves from the spinal column (the intervertebral foramen).

When there exists a possible connection between the findings of the physical examination and the neurological revelations as interpreted through the instrumentation tests the next step is the x-ray examination, but before undertaken, the chiropractor will attempt to discover the length of time that has elapsed since the person was last x-rayed or been subjected to x-ray therapy which could have increased susceptibility to radiation hazards and, in the case of a woman, whether a state of pregnancy exists. Great care is taken to protect the individual from excessive radiation. While the brief exposure attending spinal x-rays is comparatively safe as opposed to fluoroscopy and therapeutic x-rays, nevertheless, careful recording of exposure is kept and those given are well within the safety margin laid down.

If everything is relatively normal, x-ray spinographs are then taken to determine if there are any spinal misalignments, or any other pre-determined skeletal abnormalities that could cause a patient's disability. Spinographs convey vital information to the doctor of chiropractice enabling him to visualize the malposition of spinal vertebrae thereby providing the information required to re-position them.

It also tells him when a case should *not* be accepted, or subjected to spinal adjustments. Bone diseases, such as *caries fungo'sa*, tuberculosis of bone or osteolysis, for obvious reasons, come within that category as do many other types of diseases, and the patient is then advised to seek the advice of their medical doctor.

Let us take the case of a patient suffering from one or other of those two common complaints, lumbago and sciatica, which employers would probably rate to be two of the most common causes for lost working hours. Attacks of lumbago and sciatica are accompanied by the typical distortion of the spine, which produces changes of nerve impulse, causes muscles to expand and contract, and affects the normal flow of the blood stream and lymph circulation. All this affects the tonicity of the tissues.

We speak of the low-back disability primarily because attacks in that region are the most frequent, and certainly the most crippling and painful. The discs between these bones of the spine (spinal vertebrae) are the largest, and carry the larger nucleus or pulpy centre.

Contrary to the oft-expressed term "slipped disc" (this is virtually an impossibility without a fracture first occurring) these discs do not slip in, out, forward and backward, left side, right side. They are quite securely held between the adjacent vertebrae by the rim of the body of the vertebrae both above and below and surrounding muscle and ligament.

The disc is a roughly-shaped area called the Annulus and its substance is a double crescent of fibro-cartilage which contains within itself a pulpy semi-solid body which assists in presenting a cushioned pad to absorb shocks that occur involving the spine as, for instance, when one jumps over a real or imaginary obstacle, and lands heavily upon the lower extremities, feet or buttocks. (The semi-solid centre of a disc is called the Nucleus Pulposus.)

As an example of how preceding habits affecting posture of spine are involved and can affect your discs, let us suppose that your occupation involves the carrying of heavy weights (mostly on one shoulder), for example, sacks of grain, coal, or hods of bricks. In time, you develop an occupational curvature, usually sideways and forward. This compresses the discs of probably as many as five (involving seven vertebrae on this side) and in time you produce displacement of the pulpy mass to one side.

Let us now suppose that while carrying a weight on the shoulder you slip or trip over a hole, ridge, or stone, and almost fall. In trying to recover balance you put an extra severe strain and increased pressure on the pulpy mass contained within the disc. This nucleus or mass will break through the tough outer side of the disc (protrusion of the nucleus) and we have what is better known as a herniated or ruptured disc. Now, if this pulpy mass (the nucleus) does not come in contact with the nerve roots, no discomfort or symptoms will arise.

However, under suitable circumstances (such as continuing the work or strain that caused the displacement of the spinal vertebrae) this nucleus may, in a matter of hours, and sometimes as long as several days, continue its movement from its normal position and, by so doing, eventually press on the *Dura* centrally which can produce lumbago. If it reaches out still further laterally it will compress the dural extension that embraces the nerve root, producing pain in varying degrees of intensity over an area as wide as from the lower chest wall to thigh, and even as far as the knee joint. If you are unfortunate enough to get this herniation extending still further, you will in all probability suffer the painful recurrent attacks of sciatica (inflammation of the sciatic nerve). This nerve, because of its size and length of distribution, I like to think of as an extension of the spinal cord which it shares with another large nerve, the Anterior Crural Nerve, and an inflammation of one or the other of these nerves in their sheath is not only an agonizing experience, often lasting up to six weeks, but it deprives you of the last vestige of dignity in your stance and movement.

When there is a misalignment of the spinal column due to spinal vertebrae being out of rhythm with their natural position, one must correct this condition by inducing relaxation of the muscle spasm associated with it. Sometimes this can be accomplished by complete induced relaxation, such as hot baths and prolonged rest in bed.

Occasionally, too, traction may be successful, wherein an artificially induced extension of the spine permits, by the resultant suction effect, a return of the nucleus to its position within the annular disc. (This is a somewhat questionable cure-all for the painful back where there has been some degeneration of the intervertebral disc due to prolonged spinal misalignment.)

Therefore the most certain method of correction in the majority of cases is spinal adjustments, manipulation of the vertebrae by a skilled operator, your doctor of chiropractice, who, from an x-ray examination, is able to determine the exact malposition of the vertebra he is going to adjust, and who can specifically correct spinal misalignments and subluxations.

Whilst the foregoing theory of the principal causes of sciatica may be open to question when a person of fifty onwards is involved, who undoubtedly has little pulpy nucleus as compared with a person of twenty, there is much evidence that spinal adjustments, by causing a distraction of the vertebral bodies, permit the repositioning of fibrillated fragments of cartilage with subsequent relief of the painful back syndromes.

In conclusion, while I am aware of many other causes of lumbago and backache, their presence does not frequently arise in general practice, and in the unlikely event of one of these being present in your case, or if there seems to be some question of failure to respond to spinal adjustments, your doctor of chiropractice would not hesitate to call in a second opinion.

CHAPTER THREE

Medical methods of treating "Slipped Discs" compared, Whiplash and the Safety Belt, "Polio"

In the *Daily Mail* of Tuesday, 11th May 1965, an excellent article by Dr. John Anthony Parr appeared under the caption "SLIP-A-DISC Risks; and how to avoid them". It was very well written and its carefully phrased paragraphs were easily understood by the layman. It did, however, create the impression that nerve root compression between spinal vertebrae through disc distortion was only realized as a possible cause for sciatica and lumbago in 1934 and its association was made by the medical men Mixter and Barr, whereas in fact it was re-discovered by D. D. Palmer in 1895 and it was upon this basis that the science of chiropractice was established. Dr. John Anthony Parr wrote the following article:

"Thirty years ago sciatica was commonplace, all hospitals had their quota of patients attending complaining of severe pain which ran down the back of the thigh.

"Various treatments were on offer in those days. The nerve was injected with oxygen: this did no good.

"The patient was given an anaesthetic and the nerve deliberately stretched: this did no good.

"Various forms of comforting heat applications were given: these did no good.

"Failing

"And when all treatments had failed to bring relief, the orthopaedic surgeons diagnosed 'nerves' and the poor patient was sent to a psychiatrist to be 'nut shrunk'.

"Even in those days it was recognized that lumbago and sciatica often went together. And this was the position until

1934 when the medical men named Mixter and Barr put these diseases on a rational plane.

"These two men called attention to some obvious anatomical facts. That the spine consists of a number of blocks of bone called vertebrae and that in between each pair of vertebrae nature provided a shock absorber made of gristle.

"Emerging between each pair of vertebrae are a pair of spinal nerves, and Mixter and Barr's theory, so soon to be proved a fact, was that this disc of gristle could become displaced and exert pressure on one of the spinal nerves, or even a pair.

"These spinal nerves collect together to form the sciatic nerve, and if one is pressed on, the pain radiates down one or both main nerves, giving us an attack of sciatica.

"If the pressure is very severe there may be paralysis of the corresponding foot, in which case the neuro-surgeon has to operate and take out the offending disc.

"In most cases these attacks of 'slipped discs' recover with a mixture of rest, plaster casts, surgical belts or corsets and spinal traction.

"People who are out of practice should train slowly before attempting violent exercise, the rule about vigorous exercise should be 'gently, gently, catchee monkey—or else!'

"Once a spinal disc has caused trouble then in most cases the victim has to face the fact that he has a defective spine, not just one defective disc. That means he or she is liable to further attacks either with that disc, or with one of the others.

"As a preventive from further attacks the patient has to learn to sleep on a hard bed (mattress on the floor if necessary) to support the spine in a horizontal position.

"Bending

"Flexing the spine by bending has to be avoided when picking things up off the floor, and if one's last and only gold safety-pin has dropped on the floor and simply has to be retrieved, then one has to do a knees bend and sit down gracefully on the heels, keeping the spine erect while furtively feeling for the pin.

"This disorder is one of those which simply will not respond to tough determination to press on regardless of the pain.

"One has to be philosophical, take pain-relieving tablets, and rest the spine until the acute phase passes and then avoid bending the spine in the future, because if one ignores the rule suddenly when bending the disc goes again.

"Of course, if the pain is just due to lumbar fibrositis 'lumbago' then a quick manipulation which stretched the muscles will give immediate relief."

To say the least these methods are cumbersome, if not actually uncomfortable. Consider treatment by method of traction, which has been brought very much into the limelight in the last decade. Traction is an endeavour to find another method of removing vertebral compression of spinal discs. While not denying that in a very few cases traction has been of benefit, especially in cases where manipulation was contra-indicated, the personal view is that this method should not be used unless normal manipulative treatment fails to produce lasting results. When a protective posture surrounds the spine, as with a fairly rigid lumbar lordosis, if traction is applied the pressure on an affected nerve will be increased by the resultant flattening. The annulus tear may also be increased, and there will follow more pain than previously experienced.

In traction, or spinal *dis*traction therapy, the patient usually lies on a traction couch and weights are attached to the lower extremities (or if required for cervical or neck extension, to the under portion of the chin), via the usual pulley and strap attachments affixed to either or both ends of the couch. A graduated system of adding weights to the pulley is carried out as indicated, varying from 2 lbs to 5 lbs to upwards of 25 lbs to 30 lbs, or until sufficient increase of space between the vertebrae bodies has occurred to enable the nucleus protrusion to be returned to the confines of the disc proper, probably through a suction action being created. In some cases this method has to be employed for up to six or seven weeks, or even longer, during which time there is a gradual lowering of muscle tone. That is probably why a return of the condition often occurs after apparently being corrected.

We must not, however, dismiss the case for traction, or should we say spinal distraction, with a shrug of the shoulders because of

our successes without using this method. Rather let us give credit
to the doctors of medicine who have by their patient research and
endeavours brought so much light on the subject of spinal disorders to help bring relief from suffering. Not so many decades
ago, apart from surgical interference, the spine was left free from
corrections other than the relief given by long periods of rest and
pain-killing drugs.

In spinal adjustments, or manipulative therapy as practised by
the chiropractor (or more correctly, by the doctor of chiropractice) there is a difference in the method of approach from that
of the osteopath. For while the ultimate aim of both practitioners
remains the same, that is, to enable the nucleus protrusion to
return to its normal position, the chiropractor adjusts the spinal
vertebrae by hand according to instrumental and x-ray findings
of the displacement. The manipulation produces vibrations along
the spinal column and breaks up the painful muscular contraction
spasm, enabling a much quicker relief of pain to take place, and a
speedier resumption of normal bodily movements and functions.
This has been experienced time and time again. It is by no means
unusual for a patient distorted with pain and muscular spasm to
arise from the adjusting bench reasonably straight and fairly
comfortable. This applies, of course, to the ambulatory or walking
patient with a more fibrotic nucleus condition than those with
congested or turbid nucleus.

It is in the prone position that the release of the muscular spasm
following the spinal adjustment occurs. The corresponding increase in the intervertebral space permits the nucleus protrusion
to return towards its normal position within the disc. Although
it is still necessary for the patient to return for a correction of the
spinal curvature, which was the cause of the original giving-way
of the disc, he is still mobile enough to return to work without
serious loss of muscle tone due to inactivity.

Generally, the spinal column seldom occupies more than a
fleeting thought in the mind of the layman except when sharply
brought into focus during an attack of lumbago, or sciatica, or
both.

With our understanding of the mechanics of chiropractice to
this point, let us examine an effect which has become more
commonplace in present-day life when more motorists, in an

attempt at self-preservation, are adopting the use of the safety belt.

The whiplash risk, and its association with the modern so-called safety belt, was again brought to my notice in one of the daily papers. In a section dealing with motoring by Michael Kemp, the author stated that British racing motorist Graham Hill has designed a new type of car seat to stop "whiplash" which is, as he states, one of modern motoring's greatest crash risks. Whiplash is a condition that occurs when, through braking or collision with another car or reasonably solid object, the driver's or the passenger's head is violently jerked backwards, and on the recoil, as quickly thrown forwards. This can, and frequently does, tear muscles and sometimes cracks the vertebrae in the neck.

It will be remembered by some that Graham Hill, himself, became a victim of this type of disability and had to wear an inflatable surgical collar when attending the Italian Monza Grand Prix. I therefore felt that a brief article about this should be included in my book.

The doctor of chiropractice has many of these cases coming into his surgery from time to time, but there are still too many cases who succumb to this form of accident.

Just how safe is your safety belt? As we drive through the cities and countryside today we see many motorists and their passengers coming within our range of vision decorated with a broad sash of leather or some other stout fabric extending from the shoulders to the waistline, giving them the appearance of hunters journeying into the jungle after big game. The strap appears like a bandolier, and the steering wheel in the driver's hands, at a fleeting glance, looks like part of the mechanism of the sten gun of the last war.

The wearers of these strange accoutrements, with tense set faces, peer forward towards their enemy, the other folk, be they walking, or, like themselves, sitting in their vehicles, prepared to give combat to all and sundry. But with all the tension that seems to be part of the travelling act, one seems to see a smug little grin of security upon their faces as they lovingly pat the broad sash across their chest, little realizing that this body-saving device, laudable as it is, not only cannot prevent the agonizing effect of whiplash, but may serve as an additional hazard to the wearer.

By acting somewhat like a strait-jacket the safety belt immobilizes the trunk or body which normally would take part of the sudden hyperflexion and subsequent hyperextension recoil shock associated with a head-on collision, or during sudden violent breaking. We now have its effect concentrated into a small area supplied by small vertebrae such as the neck, which has no supporting structure like the ribs in the chest. In addition, to increase the hazard, we have perched atop of these smaller neck vertebrae a solid ball of ivory and brain cells which weighs on an average about seven pounds. Like a hammer head on its shaft it increases the momentum, similar to the effect produced by your "braw Scot" who demonstrates this leverage force when throwing the caber at the Highland Games.

The powerful and rapid acceleration of our modern motor-car can also produce a whiplash effect upon the passengers, who are not prepared for this sudden movement. Many a passenger has experienced the uncomfortable "snap" as the cervical neck vertebrae separate, sprain ligaments, and tear the connecting tissue between them, often causing subluxations with resultant impingement of cervical nerve roots.

Occasionally even a fracture dislocation can result from the frenzied rush and release of the clutch pedal by the motorist in his haste to reduce the time taken between two given points. This often produces disastrous results for drivers and passengers.

The majority of people who escape actual death from the violent explosive force built up between the hyperextension and hyperflexion recoil that occurs in the cervical neck, often sustain other or more permanent damage to intervertebral discs, nerve roots, and capsular structures. Sometimes meningeal branches of the spinal nerves, accompanied by haemorrhage, results from the effects of whiplash, producing swelling, stiffness and inflammation of the brachial nerves. These give rise to severe pain extending from the neck, over the shoulder, and to the elbow, which is often a prelude to the so-called "tennis-elbow", "frozen shoulder", loss of power, and the sensation of "pins and needles". Much of the above can be directly attributed to "whiplash".

As long as the internal combustion engine is there to rush us from point to point, the only way to keep down death and injury from "whiplash" is the careful driver, forever alert, considering his passengers as well as himself, by lessening speed, carefully applying his brakes, and allowing a reasonable distance in which to slow down before coming to a halt or sharp turn.

Your present safety belt, to be safe even partially, should be secured to a seat with a headrest having a restraining band of fabric, thereby preventing hyperextension and hyperflexion.

Turning from whiplash to another subject, in September 1954 the International Chiropractic Laymen's Society published an article, again by the same author, B. J. Palmer, D.D., Ph.C., under the heading *Chiropractic Principle and Practice* which gave a fairly lucid explanation of what happens during and after an attack of "polio".

The article states that *Infantile Paralysis*, commonly referred to as "polio" (Poliomyelitis) is a disease which makes its appearance usually in children. Paralysis affects muscular tissue. Other tissues of the body may be dis-eased, but only *muscular* tissue can be affected by *paralysis*, because it is the only tissue which, by shortening itself, is capable of producing movement.

Paralysis is the inability to move. Let us search for the cause of this inability by placing the affected muscle under the microscope and studying its structure. We find it discloses the same arrangement in structure as does normal muscle tissue which is capable of contracting. A most careful chemical analysis proves that muscle fibre taken from a paralysed member is identical to that taken from a normal specimen.

Let us go further and, by the use of an electric current, stimulate two specimens, one from a case of infantile paralysis and one from a normal muscle. Both tissues (for the first twelve months as a rule) react the same. Under similar conditions the ability to contract is as manifest in one as in the other.

We reach the conclusion that the reason for paralysis in muscles does not lie in abnormality in arrangement of its fibres or in elements of which it is composed. So far as science is able to determine they are the same. This conclusion is further supported by the fact that both muscle specimens will contract if supplied with proper nerve energy.

What, then, causes contraction? If there is no difference in structures of muscles which are paralysed and those which are capable of contraction, the cause must lie in mechanism upon which muscles are dependent for their contraction.

Contraction of all muscles in the body is dependent upon messages "telegraphed" to them from the brain. We decide to move our hand. Immediately following this thought power, the message is "telegraphed" to muscles of hand, and they contract. This is true of muscles in legs. Even though we may be conscious of the fact, every muscle, even those of the heart, stomach, and intestines, must receive mind messages before they can produce movement.

It is scientifically true that impelling power must originate in the brain. It is equally true that this energy must be carried to muscles before they will act. This being true, we must determine what agency is employed in transmitting these messages.;

A heavy trunk of nerve fibres extends downwards from the brain; from this trunk smaller trunks are given off at regular intervals, which finally break up and supply all parts of the body. Each kind of nerve has a special work to do. One is classed as "motor" because it serves to transmit messages from brain to muscles. The speed with which messages are carried has been proved, and today it is known that contraction in a muscle is as dependent upon the nervous system as it is upon the condition of the muscle itself.

If it is true that nothing abnormal is found in muscle tissue affected during paralysis, then we must look for a cause in some abnormality of this nervous mechanism through which contraction is controlled.

There are two ways in which this nervous tissue may be affected in cases of Paralysis.

Individual fibres may be pinched at the point where they make exit from the spine, thus decreasing carrying capacity.

Nervous tissue may be abnormal in structure to such a degree that it is incapable of transmitting messages from brain to muscles.

Examination shows that part of the nervous tissue in the spinal cord is severely inflamed in early stages of infantile paralysis. Following this inflammation there is a hardening of some tissues in the cord, and a change in its structure. (If this condition remains the same, carrying ability of the nerves is permanently affected because the brain, spinal cord, and nerve fibres are supplied by nerves which carry life currents essential to their normal function.)

CHAPTER FOUR

Nerve Impulses,
The Anatomy of the Spinal Column, Pain

Man being the animal that he is, unwilling to conform to a fixed pattern of living, unwilling to content himself, "as the other animals do", to just being himself, eating, drinking, sleeping and procreating, restlessly surges through his life span, doing more than he was built to do, wishing to be still more than he is, rushes through the air at a fantastic speed, travelling overland at often more than a hundred miles an hour and in his struggles through life he twists, distorts, dislocates and fractures his bony framework as he explores the depths of the ocean, the heights of the mountains, the labyrinth passages underground, and in so doing creates spinal cord compression within the neural canal especially within the "foramen magnum", the circular base of skull through which passes the spinal cord.

This spinal cord contains the accumulation of multiple extensional brain fibres which it carries from brain to every tissue cell. Its passage is downwards through each successive bony ring (vertebra) between each of which is a cartilage mass, or disc to cushion the shock man's spine is subjected to, and this it does well. However, due to the abnormal strain, posture, shock through accidents due to his unnatural manner of living, these discs suffer compression, distortion, and rupture, and the effect is interference with nerve distribution from nerve root outward to tissue cells.

At every inter-vertebral space situated laterally between each two vertebrae are openings through which nerves emit from the spinal cord, passing externally outwards to each muscle, organ, and tissue cell. When through accident, concussion of force, or continued postural strain a vertebra distorts the inter-vertebral space it reduces the opening and at times impairs nerve distribution, often resulting in reduced frequency of muscular rhythm which could reduce or destroy function.

It is therefore necessary to remove or correct any condition where there exists disc interference, to restore the health of mankind suffering from this type of disability, sometimes medically through rest, body belts, plaster casts and traction, or chiropractically through "vertebral manipulations", better known as spinal adjustments.

As emphasis is constantly being placed upon diagnosis by the medical profession, it sometimes becomes a little difficult for the general public to understand why the doctor of chiropractice is always talking in terms of analysis and adjustments when discussing dis-ease and diabilities, and their correction by spinal adjustments.

Now Dorland's Medical Dictionary defines—

"Diagnosis" as "The art of distinguishing one disease from another"

"Analysis" as "A separation of component parts"

"Disease" as "A definite morbid process having a characteristic train of symptoms"

"Symptom" as "any evidence of disease or of a patient's condition".

The medical diagnostician, by questioning and by the use of diagnostic equipment gathers a group of symptoms or effects and names that group of effects, epilepsy, cirrhosis and cancer of the liver, tumours, and so on, after which, the physician prescribes treatment for the effects which is the proper procedure, if one is to concentrate only on the effects of a cause.

The Chiropractic doctor is concerned with cause, and his education, equipment, and work, is with the cause of effects; not with the effects or symptoms. The Chiropractic doctor must know what is the cause, its location, what produces it, and how best to remove it.

In a great many of these cases he finds, with his knowledge and his instruments, a vertebral interference affecting the transmission of vital energy between brain and body, and having located this cause he proceeds to make the necessary corrections (adjustments) to reduce and eventually eliminate the effects when possible.

Webster's dictionary interpretation of *adjust* is to make exact, to fit, to make correspondent or comfortable, to bring into proper relation.

An adjustment, therefore, chiropractically, is the name of the action made by him when he adjusts into proper relation "innate intelligence" to bring into line the *mental* with its equivalent physical body. We are not merely affecting the subluxated vertebra when we adjust it, but every atom of the human system. It is impossible to estimate the number of vibrations to the second required to keep the blood corpuscle in motion. Imagine, then, the rapidity with which a sensation travels on its course when it affects every neuron, ganglion and plexus of the entire neurological system.

It is estimated that the heart lifts an average weight of 20 lbs to every throb. In the adult being the heart beats on an average 70 times per minute, 60 minutes per hour, and 24 hours a day. This means an average lift of actual weight of 84,000 lbs per hour, or 2,016,000 lbs per day. What, then, must be the jar to the molecular "building" in which we live, when a thrust or adjustment is given upon any one segment of the spinal column?

Accepting this reasoning it is self-evident that we do something more than merely place a subluxated vertebra in alignment. We have not only released the impinged nerve at the subluxated point, or to put it another way, opened a valve to let loose the flow of life, but by the thrust made, produced a concussion of molecular energy coursing through every minute part of our anatomy at a speed that cannot be measured. This being true, think what an adjustment may do to the nerve terminals of our electrified structure.

Many patients who have undergone long periods of disability and sickness find a great reduction in function often accompanied with wasting of tissue. They are surprised when an aching part or parts of the body develop a fairly sharp pain during the early stages of recovery. We are frequently asked "Why do I have pain returning, when to all intents and purposes function is improving?"

Before answering this question in some detail, we must study the spinal system.

A well balanced healthy spine, housing—as it does—the spinal cord with its contingent of nerve roots conveying vital nerve forces to most of the organs and parts of the body through the Intervertebral Foramina (openings on either side of the spinal vertebra) is essential to maintain a healthy body, and therefore the following information should be studied.

The spinal column is a flexible accumulation of vertebrae (irregularly shaped segments of bone) of which there are twenty-six, twenty-four true vertebrae, that is, movable segments, and two false, the latter being named the Sacrum and Coccyx.

Commencing from the first segment, which joins the head at its base (the occipital bone) and counting downwards, the first seven form the spine of the neck, and are called *Cervical vertebrae*. They should form a forward curve (concave forward) terminating between the upper section of the shoulders.

The next twelve are called *Dorsal* or *Thoracic vertebrae*, the uppermost of them forming a natural curve upwards and backwards (convex).

Now we have the five *Lumbar vertebrae*, forming an anterior concavity, that is a forward direction.

All the above are balanced upon the base of the Sacrum (the upper part) which forms the posterior (spinal) portion of the *Pelvis*, together with the remaining four *Sacral vertebrae*. The lowest, or fifth, forms the apex of the true Sacrum which is joined below by the rudimentary tail bones (Cauda), the four bones being known as the Coccyx.

In childhood, both the sacrum and the coccyx contain separate segments (separated by hyaline certilage) the sacrum containing five and the coccyx four, but in adult life they ossify together forming a Sacral section (five segments joined together) and a coccygeal one (four sections joined together) but at times again separated by injury. The adult, therefore, has twenty-four true vertebrae and two false (Sacrum and Coccyx). So in effect the child has more bones in the back (33) than the adult, who only has 26.

Anatomists refer to the *spine* as being the movable vertebrae (excluding the Sacrum and Coccyx). The *spinal column* on the other hand is from twenty-seven inches to twenty-eight-and-three-quarters. On average, the length of the *spine*—twenty-three inches—is about one-third the total height of the individual, and the male spine three inches longer than the female.

If we look at the spinal column from the side we are aware of the double anterior and posterior curves; roughly the neck bends forward, the upper dorsals backwards, the lowest dorsals and lumbars again bend forward, the base (upper part of the Sacrum) tilts backwards, following by a forward bending of the Sacral apex and the Coccyx.

These natural curves add greatly to the strength of the spine and, in addition, add beauty to the human form.

The spinal column is very adaptive to weight distribution, and the more one section goes forwards or backwards, so another section adapts itself in the opposite direction; this is especially true during the changes incurred during such conditions as pregnancy, abdominal tumours, and obesity.

An increase of an anterior curve during pregnancy is not known as an abnormality but a compensation, equalizing the weight distribution, and a re-adaption should take place. But if, for any reason, this re-adaption does not occur, the curve could increase and then become a curvature, the cause of which must be found and corrected by spinal adjustments.

Another function of the spinal curves is that of absorbing the shock or jarring effect taken by the spine when a person jumps down from a height. If, during a fall, the whole weight of the body were taken at the Sacral and Coccygeal extremity, instead of some of the shock being absorbed within the curves of the spine, there would follow considerable damage to the spinal cord, and possibly the brain.

The spinal column holds the body erect, supports the head, and provides an anchorage for the ribs which, in turn, form the bony cage that protects and contains the heart, lungs, liver, upper portion of the stomach, and, at the back, the kidneys. In addition, it holds the weight of the body and transmits some of this weight to the pelvis. With the normal flexible consistency of the spine it permits all bodily movements such as extension and counter-extension, flexion, and rotation.

The spine, therefore, is the focal point for all parts of the body which are *directly or indirectly* attached to it.

By far the most vital function of the spinal column is its use in housing the spinal cord, and its protection within its bony column, for life itself depends upon this. It is through minor, and sometimes major, subluxations, luxations, and dislocations of the spinal segments (the vertebrae) that we are able to trace some of the major diseases and disabilities of the body.

Try and visualize the brain as a vast power station, housed in that solid block of ivory known as the head. Follow its transmission of nerve force, motor, sensory and intelligence, through the opening in the base of the skull (known as the *foramen magnum*), which sends out the waves from that broadcasting house of yours, to and through the various channels which are to be found between the junction of each of the vertebra.

Directly attached to the brain, the spinal cord conveys these nerve impulses down the spinal column, pairing off between each vertebra, on its downward course supplying, first in the neck region, impulses to the brachial nerves; it supplies functional needs to the arms; a little lower it pairs off further impulses to heart, bronchial tubes, lungs, and other organs. It continues the distribution next to the liver, solar plexus, and for stomach needs; on to diaphragm, kidneys, small and large intestines, contents of the pelvis, reproductive organs, and bladder.

The spinal cord then divides into branches, running down both legs, great and lesser sciatic nerves, crural nerves, and so on. Each impulse conveyed stimulates circulation, tells which muscles to flex or extend in order to produce movement; then, on its return journey, it sends messages back through the cord, advising the brain when our shoes are too tight, our feet too cold, and like matters. That is why we must keep these channels open by correcting any bony or cartilage changes that prevent these messages getting through. That is chiropractic function, and the reason for its doctors.

Atlas, Axis and Occipital articulations when not in juxtaposition, produce compression of the spinal cord in that region. Patients think pain comes from the region where they are conscious of painful symptoms, but this is not always so. The painful nerves (as sometimes occurs in sciatica) may be inflamed through pressure in the upper cervical region (top spinal vertebrae) and could travel down to the point of leaving the spinal column, creating discomfort to the terminal point of nerve sensitivity.

Cord pressure in the upper spine may be produced by subluxations of Atlas or Axis in such a way as actually to reduce the size of the foramina (Magnum Foramen) especially by a side-slipping of the Atlas (first vertebra) to one side and forward or by a body pivot of Axis. If the check ligaments that hold the Odontoid in position (a process of the axis vertebra, have been subjected to severe strain as for example during the sudden braking of a car creating a whiplash forward thrust of head and neck vertebrae, the Odontoid process may also be responsible for some of the reduction of space in the Foramina.

Other portions of the spine can have misalignments, but rarely compress emitting nerves direct, owing to the interlocking pedicles, although constant misalignment can create changes in the disc causing nucleus protrusion that can, when inflamed, squeeze the surrounding tissue of the nerves at that point.

Originally a person has normal healthy organs and tissue with normal feeling and has no pain or sensation of it, but a vertebral subluxation interferes with normal feeling and produces pain on the declining side. This continues until a state of limited or no feeling or no function occurs.

A correction (adjustment) of this subluxation restores function, feeling is then on the incline, and increased feeling produces *constructive* pain until function is normal.

Your Chiropractor discriminates between pain on the declining side, and between pain on the incline back to normal pre-subluxation health. All that the unfortunate patient knows is that he suffers *pain*. He wants to get rid of it, complains about getting worse, and wants to take "something" to kill pain. If pain is killed by drugs, when the condition is actually on the upgrade, this would prevent neurocalometer or neurocalograph accurate readings and stop the patient getting well, through failure to detect pressure interference.

It is easy to kill pain. Medically it is done with many drugs, which is to be commended in emergencies and accidents but continued use may give a false sense of comfort and, at times, permit disease to progress to a state where a condition becomes so chronic because of the patient's *ease* that it is sometimes impossible to arrest.

An example of pain towards recovery is when an arm or leg "goes to sleep". One has no pain, no feeling, no function. Pressure on the arm or leg is released and pain is experienced as "pins and needles". This is the upgrade to normal feeling, normal sensation, and normal function.

When friction on any part of the body is constantly applied, nature protects these vital parts by building up callous tissue. In the case of prolonged friction, in the upper cervical (neck) region as in a side-slip of Atlas, or inferiority of Axis, or both, nature protects the spinal cord by similar tissue covering. If this continues, there is a possibility of its producing its own reduction of the space for the passage of the spinal cord. This pressure, therefore, could continue for some months and sometimes even years after the vertebral subluxations are corrected.

Likewise nature produces *ankylosis* (abnormal consolidation of a joint) and *exostosis* (an abnormal outgrowth of bone from the surface of it) to protect regions from the continual strain of spinal misalignments. These will remain there until Innate Intelligence decides that this support or protection is no longer necessary.

One quite frequently finds that a person who has suffered discomfort for years owing to spinal misalignment suddenly has it modified to a great degree, and again it disappears altogether. This is especially true of the person who is approaching the pensionable age group. In my opinion, the change of spinal balance due to the reduction of the discs between the vertebrae, can ease the pressure at one point, relieving the compression of the annular disc to such an extent that the necessity for supporting ankylosis or exostosis is no longer required and in time will disappear. It is a fact that one loses height in the declining age group through this process of reduction of depth of intervertebral discs.

Just as we frequently hear of people suddenly becoming unable to see or hear or losing the use of some of their limbs. due to a sudden shock or concussion of force to the body so, on the other side of the case book, we find a restoration to normal following such shock applications.

Many years ago, in the first few years of my practice in Canada, a case of this kind occurred to a prospective patient of mine. She was a woman in the middle forties who suffered from a paralysis of the lower extremities. She had been thoroughly examined and x-rayed, and was given a further appointment when the result of the x-ray spinograph was to be explained to her.

On the day reserved for this purpose, and about an hour after her appointment time, my receptionist received a telephone call to say that she would not be keeping the appointment as the ambulance which was conveying her had swerved to avoid a fast-moving fire engine. The strain on the ambulance had opened the rear doors and the patient was thrown to the road. When assisted to her feet she found not only could she stand, but also walk a little.

Later that day I called on her and asked if she would permit me to re-x-ray her, which was done a few days later. Upon comparison with the first set of plates (which showed subluxated vertebrae in the upper cervical spine) it was found that this appeared corrected, together with a left lateral misalignment of the lumbar vertebrae, again proving that this accidental concussion of force had corrected the spinal condition.

While this case had a successful "adjustment", I do not suggest that you should risk such a method of correction, as there is no guarantee that it will always work! It does prove, however, that a concussion of force on vertebrae which are out of alignment will activate muscles and surrounding tissue to restore the vertebrae to their origial position. Conversely, it could create, and undoubtedly frequently does produce, the first subluxations.

Needless to say, I kept a watchful eye on this case for nearly twelve months, because I am not impressed by patients' exclamations that this or that is better after only a few visits. Occasionally a patient's reserve energy, plus a great deal of optimism, will work apparent miracles, but I prefer the test of time as to its permanence, and I am pleased to say this patient passed such a test.

Remember, one cannot give chiropractice "a trial"; one must have the entire spinal nerve distribution normal to produce health, and this frequently takes time.

CHAPTER FIVE

Drugs and their Misuse

Cases suffering from pain, who cannot sleep, take drugs to kill pain or produce sleep. When they do this they little realize that they are doing the very thing which eventually defeats the ultimate objective—health. Opiates, narcotics, and hypnotics, do bring about immediate cessation of pain or production of sleep, but the effect is always temporary. At the same time the use of drugs deadens the flow of mental impulses and feeling.

Drugs are frequently used to create a type of happiness. Only happiness in the true sense can produce healthiness. Anxiety produces stresses which set up tension in the nervous system. A combination of tensions will create a muscle spasm or cramp which, in turn, reduces the circulation and causes tissue compression. When such tissue surrounds vital motor or sensory nerves it produces a condition of inflammation which affects the nerves within their sheaths. The result is pain, loss of motion, dulling of sensation, or all three.

In turn, the contractions result in uneven pressures on the spinal system leading to distortion and uneven distribution of bodily weight, which in itself produces further pain. Pressure may be exerted on one side of the annular disc to cause the nucleus or centre of the disc to be forced to its opposite side. After the nucleus has been in this position for some time, a sudden strain in an awkward position of sufficient severity can force the nucleus or central pulpy mass of the disc through the intervertebral disc which is then herniated or ruptured. Chiropractors call this effect the nuclear protrusion which is often erroneously called a "slipped disc". In the case of an actual slipped disc there exists a fracture-dislocation.

When we have a rupture of the annular disc the nerve roots are compressed with the same accompanying pain, loss of motion, and sensation, according to the severity which is produced in the case of cramp. There is nothing that the patient can do about this condition except to call in a specialist who will make the necessary adjustments to return the vertebrae to their normal position where possible. This is all that the doctor of chiropractice aims to do. Innate Intelligence, which you may prefer to call instinct or subconscious mind, does the rest to restore you to health and happiness.

You can, however, do a great deal to prevent the tension and discomfort produced by anxiety and stress by not getting worked up by every bit of news relative to your body that you read or hear about. Try to take a sane view of all the news, views, and forebodings brought within your orbit, sometimes by thunderous sound effects on radio and television, and by those warnings received in the lecture hall, soap box in the park, or in heavy print on the news sheet.

These few examples should suffice:

If you drink alcohol you will probably die of cirrhosis of the liver.
Fatty foods cause heart disease.
Hot baths remove the natural oils from your body making you subject to colds.
Butter introduces too much cholesterol into the arteries, producing arterial sclerosis and heart bloc,

and only a few months ago it was pointed out that:

Keeping your bedroom windows open while sleeping was probably another cause of bronchitis or lung disease.

After all these warning cries, which are in themselves causes of mental stress, we are solemnly told that stress causes ulcers. Small wonder that people think that everything they enjoy is a potential killer, illegal, immoral, or fattening.

One can have a sound heart, lungs, liver, stomach, and still be sick because you have acquired the modern disease "Chronic Anxiety". Naturally you would be foolish to smoke if you are an asthmatic, have coronary thrombosis, or stomach ulcers, and again, you would be equally foolish to consume alcohol regularly if you have gout, liver trouble, extemely high blood pressure, or ulcers, or if your physician advises you to abstain because of some unidentified disability. Apart from these reasons for abstaining, alcohol with moderation, say a few ounces per day, is still the safest tranquillizer, and if taken immediately before retiring is the best sleep producer of them all, unlike drugs, that can build up a dangerous accumulation of chemical matter in the body if taken beyond the short period any wise medical practitioner prescribes. It produces no thalidomide babies, depression, delusions of persecution, suicidal impulses, or other undesirable side-effects, and as a tension reducer can often be valuable in some heart and artery diseases.

The voice of medical doom on TV, radio, and press, is fast making us a nation of hypochondriacs, and while no one should be fool enough to ignore the warnings of their physicians, be they medical, chiropractic, osteopathic, natureopathic, or any other specialized health service beings, you must not adopt diseases forecast for you by the modern news dispenser, or you will soon be beyond help.

So many people today are forever checking this little pain, or that little discomfort, against the symptoms they hear or read about as being associated with this or that disease.

Fear creates an anxiety complex so vivid that they are unable to enjoy life even when the little ache, pain, or distress symptoms are absent. In my lifetime I have seen the attitudes of people and their living habits change so much through warnings about this disease, or that, being brought to their notice by press and magazine, sometimes accompanied by advertisements of this or that drug on the same page to relieve the real or imaginary ailment they have just read about.

You cannot sleep, so you swallow this or that tranquillizer. The next morning you feel unable to tackle the day's work, so you take some pep pills to overcome the drug-induced lethargic state. You read again that your real or imaginary ailments may be caused by vitamin deficiency, so you add to the collection of little bottles you carry around all day one that contains vitamins A to E.

Your nerves are sedated, pepped up, fed with this hormone or the vitamins you buy from your chemists, and the ordinary functions that nature intended us to use, to live, love, and be happy with, are so confused, that they reduce or give up their activities within our body and mind.

I am not suggesting that you discontinue taking the prescription recommended by your family physician. At least he knows what he wishes to add or withhold from your daily requirements when you are sick, but rather that you discontinue being your own diagnostician when it involves the use of drugs. This is your doctor's responsibility, and in his wisdom he will soon take you off them when the crisis is past, but if through overwork he forgets, you would be wise to ask when you may leave off the prescription, otherwise you could build up an accumulation of drugs that could be detrimental to your health.

One must remember there is no known drug that can specifically replace a vertebral subluxation, malposition, or misalignment, and if your enforced rest cure for so-called slipped disc does not by time and relaxation cure your lumbago, sciatica, or other conditions that originate from vertebral malposition within ten to fourteen days, you should visit a specialist who knows how to re-position them by hand.

Should you choose a doctor of chiropractice to correct the vertebral misplacement that is the possible cause of your disability, it will be of material assistance to his spinal analysis if you refrain from taking opiates, narcotics and hypnotics for at least twenty-four hours before the appointment. In taking drugs, while they create a temporary relief from pain and produce sleep, they also deaden the efferent flow of mental impulses and the afferent flow of impressions to the point of deadening feeling.

This interferes with neurocalometer readings taken by the doctor of chiropractice as also is the case with other users of thermo recording instruments. It is essential that the spinal specialist locates the exact position of vertebral displacement where there is nerve root involvement, but if through the deadening of function and sensation the thermo-couple detectors fail to register this part, then, although a vertebral subluxation can exist, and interference with normal nerve transmission be present, your chiropractor would be unable to help as he must have proof of its existence.

Take a normal body, feed it drugs, and you will paralyse sensitivity and function. The body will lose feeling as well as motion.

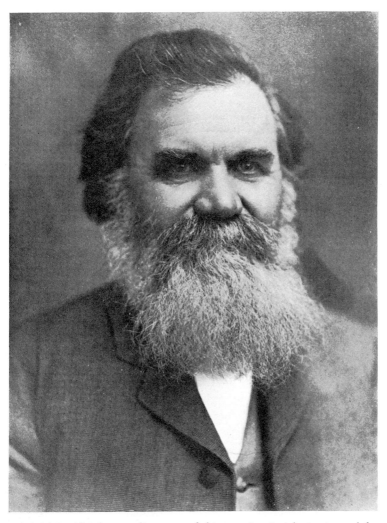

1. Daniel David Palmer, rediscoverer of chiropractic principles in 1895 and the founder of modern Chiropractice.

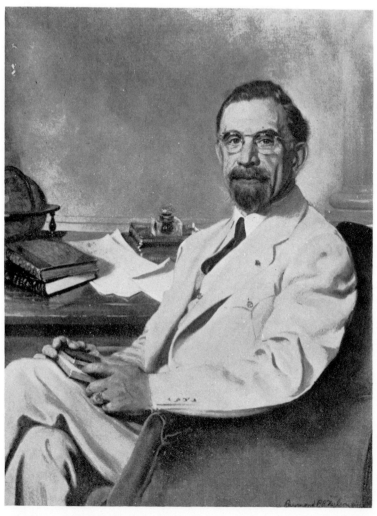

2. Bartlett Joshua Palmer, D.C., Ph.C., developer of Chiropractice and President of the first Chiropractic College, 1906–1961.

If that happens with normal healthy bodies, how much more does it happen when a person is sick or below par!

Chiropractors rely on their instruments to determine the location of nerve interference and warn their patients not to take anything which will interfere, maintaining that it is better to suffer *one day* without drugs than to suffer years with them.

With the information gained from both the neurocalograph and spinograph (x-ray of spine) the chiropractor can make a specific directional thrust upon the subluxated or mis-aligned vertebra, thereby releasing any pressure on nerve roots caused by such malpositions. This permits the restoration of normal quantity flow of mental impulses to the body, at the same time relieving the brain of some of the pressure caused by the damming back of nerve energy, when its expression is reduced by interference, and a restoration of normal function follows.

We now have an increase from below normal to normal nerve force, which reaches the periphery or distal ends of those nerves in the body tissue cells or body organs, and results in their increased action. After making due allowance for repair and development, which requires time, we reach a condition of "ease" or health.

Many teenagers and quite a few adults seem to find it impossible to go through any normal day's work or play without fortifying themselves with either vitamins, pep pills, or at times, tranquillizers. In the Americas especially, and in a slightly lesser degree France, then England, it is fast becoming a normal procedure for people to instinctively reach out for the bottle of vitamins or pep pills as soon as they are awake, without stopping to ask themselves if they really do need them. In the majority of cases they do not bother to consult their doctor first to find out whether they are beneficial or harmful, nor do they question whether the constant use of them is producing a build-up of harmful side-effects.

It appears that a great number of adults started taking extra vitamins in pill or tablet form as a result of reading or listening to advertisements claiming that this or that vitamin relieved fatigue, produced manly vitality, protected you from colds; and while there is no foundation in fact for these claims, nevertheless if a vitamin consumer managed to avoid a cold during a poor summer or a bad winter, he would immediately attribute this to the extra vitamins he consumed, and in many cases he would take them for life, notwithstanding the fact that he probably lived in the best-fed country on earth.

In such a country it is difficult to buy food that is not already rich in vitamins, and while the consumption of extra vitamins does not do any damage, except to the bank balance, it does commence a habit of pill dosing oneself without knowledge or guidance, for in truth, there is not five per cent of the average population who could give an intelligent answer to the questions: What are vitamins? Which group comes from which source of supply? or How do you know what vitamins you lack?

Your self-medicating adult next starts taking a few pep pills "just to tide them over a busy day at the office" or as a boost before meeting their partners at home, or just as a "lift" before stepping out for the evening.

Teenagers frequently take pep pills in one form or another because it gives them a false sense of security when sitting for exams, applying for a position, or just to boost themselves up for yet another night out, when, in reality, they require an occasional early night to repair the damage of too many nights out.

Frequently teenagers take pep pills, or to quote their own jargon "Goof balls", because others in their particular group use them, and they do not like to be called "Chicken" or admit that they are not (as they are so fond of saying) "with it" and, like the addicted adult, most of them think the pills are harmless, and are thrilled by the sense of elation, extra energy, and false power, often accompanied by acts of foolish aggressiveness that follows this pepping up process.

If they would only learn that pep pills, instead of being harmless, are responsible for numerous crimes, many with violence, and a vast number of accidents frequently involving a number of innocent people can be traced to the "pepped up" vehicle driver.

One of the main reasons why "pep pills" cause so many "inexplicable accidents" while motoring is probably the sudden "let down" experienced by the driver when the effect of the drug wears off.

Many drivers take pep pills to boost themselves up when driving long distances "to prevent sleepiness", and if they are already tired before completion of the journey, will resort to an increased number of pills which invigorates and stimulates an already tired body, then suddenly, with no warning, comes the "let down"—overpowering IRRESISTIBLE FATIGUE—causing loss of control of the vehicle, with injury, often fatal, following for the driver and, all too often, innocent people.

In concluding this chapter, mention must be made about the use of tranquillizers, for whilst these are amongst the newer forms of sedatives, and not nearly as frequently used as vitamins or pep pills, they still should not be used except under the direction of your family physician, and even then, never take any form of tranquillizers if you are under the influence of alcohol as the combination of these has been known to have fatal consequences.

Should you feel the need for tranquillizers in order to meet your business requirements, then you are either not suited to such emotional and exacting conditions of responsibility, or you are lacking the assets of good well-balanced food, do not lead a normal physically active life, meaning sport or exercise promoting the active movement of the principal muscles of the body such as walking, swimming, golf, tennis, etc., or suitable hobbies requiring much bodily movement, and lastly, possibly insufficient sleep.

Should you still feel below par, not able to cope with your business, consult your doctor, have a good physical check up, and let him tell you which, if any, vitamins your body is short of.

Have a spinal analysis made by a reputable doctor of chiropractice to be certain there is no interruption with the normal transmission of nerve energy from brain through spinal cord, the adjacent nerve roots and nerves to the organs and parts of the body.

On no account join the army of people indulging in self-medication. It is often harmful, and could result in premature death.

CHAPTER SIX

Mental and Physical Attitude to Health and Activity at Middle Age

Many people get the idea that they must live with their ailments because of their age. They are inclined to accept general lassitude; bouts of depression; irritability, accompanied many times by headaches; an inability to concentrate and to converse intelligently with those around them; and all the little aches—real or imaginary —that make their lives a misery, or worse still, make life a misery for those around them.

Many have the commonsense to go to their physician for advice and treatment. Undoubtedly some do respond to a tonic especially if, after the examination, they have been assured that there is nothing really wrong with them. On occasion the physician is puzzled by the absence of any apparent cause for the patient's condition, and occasionally uses the phrase "You must learn to live with it". Then we have the sorry spectacle of seeing a good business man, or a happy working man, drooping around the house in a state of apathy or self-pity, neither of which is conducive to good companionship.

Many times they are pushed into our surgeries by relatives or friends. In a good many cases, it is possible to trace the cause of their disabilities to an interference with the direct flow of nerve force normally transmitted from the brain to all parts of the body through the medium of the spinal cord. In a high percentage of these cases, we find the interference caused by vertebral subluxations, especially in the upper cervical spine. After a period of time, during which corrective adjustments are made to the spine by an efficient doctor of chiropractice, the patient again becomes an alert, active, member of society.

There is nothing miraculous about this transformation if we remember that no part of the human body can function normally if deprived of nerve energy sufficient for its task.

I have found, that, where the spinal cord or nerve roots emitting from it are subject to compression interference and spinal manipulations are indicated, age has little to do with recovery, except that, of course, a little more time is required. One must remember that spinal adjustments are possible, with very good results, at all age levels.

With the assistance of the x-rays, we are able to detect unhealthy bone structures, and spinal adjustments are not made in such cases. Great care is taken when there is a suspicion of abnormal brittleness of bone, but it is not true, as many people believe, that all bones become brittle with old age. Whilst heavy adjustment of the spinal column is contra-indicated at any age, light spinal adjustments skilfully applied by a trained chiropractic doctor. carry no age limits or discomfort, and are undoubtedly an aid to longevity.

Many people who are able and fit at eighty and ninety owe their lives, health, and activity to men like Pasteur, Lister, Banting, on the medical side, and to D. D. Palmer, re-discoverer of the art and science of chiropractice, on the other. I think it more than a coincidence that 1895 brought the discovery of x-radiation by Roentgen, and the re-discovery of the chiropractic science. The former was just as necessary in specific detection of the vertebral position in man to enable corrective spinal adjustments to be made.

It is frequently demonstrated that there are vast reserves of energy stored within us, both in reasoning power and vitality that enables even frail crippled persons to overcome their general apathy and call upon reserves of vitality that they never realized existed until an emergency arose. An invalid, trapped within a burning building, can draw upon such a reserve by the action of the brain sending urgent messages over the network of nerves, stimulating and energizing glands and blood vessels into increased activity according to the need (regardless of age group) making it possible for that person to get away some distance, before falling down in a state of collapse.

It seems that Hormones are released at such times, making possible activity capable of dealing with situations far beyond our ordinary requirements. In other words the sum total of physical and chemical processes are stepped up to meet emergencies.

A great part of these reserves of vital nerve force could, of course, be prevented from functioning should we have an interference with nerve distribution, by compression of nerve roots through vertebral subluxations affecting the source of supply.

This is why spinal adjustments become necessary, from time to time, to release interference with nerve function, restore normal circulation, and promote activity of both motor and sensory nerves that make mobility possible.

Patients undergoing spinal adjustments for some physical disability or limitation of movement, are sometimes surprised to find, on checking with their family physician, that their abnormally high or low blood pressure has returned nearly to normal, and heart symptoms have reduced, and at times, magically disappeared and are always much more tolerable. But this is not particularly remarkable. It is merely a question of body mechanics becoming adjusted to permit normal functioning once again.

Your doctor of chiropractice never regards abnormal blood pressure as a disease in itself, merely as the inevitable and sometimes beneficial effect of some resistance in the body. This causes the heart to work harder to overcome such resistance and get the blood through these distressed areas which otherwise would be deprived of this life-giving stream. Spinal adjustments release body tension, and allow pressure to return to normal . With a drop in tension, there automatically follows a drop in resistance. In other words, if you clear obstruction, you permit free flow. Tension produces resistance, and this obstructs circulation.

Similarly, men and women suffering from disease of the heart derive great benefit from the release of nerve force which follows spinal vertebral correction. With the restoration of normal nerve force, we restore normal blood supply, which in turn brings about healthy muscle tonicity within the heart itself, restoring vigour, and easing restriction within the chest wall.

This may be described as nerve and mechanical factors reducing tension, for tension is an anxiety state which produces contraction of muscle and tissue. It can therefore be understood that a relaxed approach to living, plus a normal spinal balance, and the absence of any interference with both nerve and blood distribution can maintain tranquillity and perfect health.

Many people who have become mentally ill through emotional

or business worries, which in turn produced anxiety tension, muscular contractions, and interference with nerve distribution, have been extremely grateful for the recovery of their normal, full brain activity, and in many cases, release from their voluntary entry into institutions, through having spinal conditions corrected, principally constriction of the upper cervical spine.

We are all faced with the fact that, compared with fifty years ago, man's expectation of life has risen very considerably. We should, therefore, be prepared to work longer, live more vitally, and enjoy the fruits of our labour, not by sitting back and contemplating them, but by planning and creating more exciting things to do in the future. For if this extra span of life continues, and I believe it will increase still further, we will have to postpone that planned retirement and put our back into work again.

As you look at many of the people around it will be obvious to you, as it is to me, that middle age does not begin at 30 as it did fifty years ago for women, and at 40 for men. We now find women looking 30 at 50, and men enjoying youthful activities at 60 or even 70. Middle age today is around 50 for both sexes, and old age just begins around the 70's with expectation of health and enjoyment up to the 80's.

I have very many patients of well over 80 who are clear in brain and still enjoying a good day's work. This makes me believe that man is as old as his spine, for when that is kept supple and free from vertebral subluxations he can enjoy life to the full.

The prematurely old are those who are ever conscious of middle age. They sit looking aimlessly about their surroundings and seem to take on a lack-lustre appearance as they slowly roll their hands together, which lie in their laps, seemingly seeking some excuse for their inactivity. One can almost hear them saying to themselves "Well, I suppose I must expect this and that at my time of life" and adopting the "I will have to learn to live with it" attitude of complacency. Their minds wander further in contemplation as they think they are up against that period known as the "change of life".

We have many of these pre-aged men and women literally pushed into our surgeries by their enlightened relatives or friends, and shortly, the reaction of these people to the correction of spinal imbalance becomes evident to us, and brings much of the joy and feeling of worthwhileness to those who are privileged to practise the science and art of chiropractice. They start to walk with a firm stride, have a new light in their eyes, and a zest for living and working. They become aware of the wonders around them, feeling new energy surging through them following the release of pressure interference with nerve distribution after the correction of spinal imbalance by adjustments of vertebral subluxations.

We now know that spinal adjustments can release a trigger mechanism which stimulates neuro-endoctrine nerve gland activity and that as a result of this, adrenalin, sympathin, and other vital fluids are poured into circulating blood. It is as simple as that.

One of the most common disorders of middle age is the so-called lumbago. However, we find that only a small percentage of those patients presenting themselves for chiropractic adjustments are genuine lumbago cases. The majority of low-back disorders, and the fashionably known prolapsed intervertebral disc, appear to be caused by *sacro-iliac* strain of more or less severity which may spread upwards from the sacro-iliac dimple, through the lumbar region, and result in inflammation of the sciatic nerve root. This latter is accompanied by a marked muscular spasm in which the spine is drawn to one side and the patient is unable to flex or extend his back, and with movement from one position to another very limited by pain.

At times we find cases hesitant to have spinal adjustments when they have a severe painful back condition, thinking that such adjustments would be too painful. But I can assure them that the light adjustments made to regions much higher than the specifically painful one will release the muscle spasm and produce relief from pain very quickly. In many cases a marked return to the normal upright position is effected before leaving the surgery.

Further visits are necessary to correct all the spinal displacements, and the patient is encouraged to exercise, resume work as soon as possible, and thus avoid losing muscular tonicity which is so vital to the spinal column to maintain its erect position.

In closing this chapter, which has been written mainly for the middle-age group, I would like to suggest that unless specifically advised to the contrary by your physician, you get down to systematic bodily activity, especially walking, which increases your pulse rate, oxygen intake, and the elimination of waste products, particularly through the pores of the skin, and sweat glands.

And lastly, that heart of yours. Too many people express fear and concern when they become aware of a little extra chest thump. They seem to have an idea that the heart must maintain an even tick-tock like a clock, and that anything exceeding this is a sign of impending doom. Then follows that "fear and apprehension" that strikes so many among the middle-aged.

Much more time should be devoted to instructing humans about the potential power and function of the heart. They should be made to realize that it is the strongest organ in the body and that an occasional burst of energy resulting in a stronger, more rapid pulse rate for a short period of time, increases the elasticity of the heart muscles and, in addition, by temporarily forcing more blood through, thereby stretches the walls of the arteries and creates more elasticity therein. The tendency for deposits of hard fat and cholesterol to adhere to the walls of the arteries is considerably reduced with less tendency to heart or artery bloc.

So, get your walking clothes on and stride forth into the great outside. Bring back that glow to your cheeks, that light in your eyes, and the good clear chest that you had before you slumped into that easy chair of yours where your only exercise was turning the knobs of the radio or television set. You will feel years younger, your family and friends will be delighted to see that paunch disappear, and that old friendly greeting will make you once again someone worth knowing.

Since writing this chapter it was interesting to note in the *Sunday Express* on 1st October 1967 an article written by Robert Chapman entitled "Science and You". "Soon life may be six-score years and five"—he wrote. "Many of today's children and a fair proportion of their parents are likely to live to 80 or 90 and enjoy it.

"For the average age limit in technologically advanced countries is going up steadily, doctors say.

"Already indeed doctors claim that they have provided us with a medical blueprint for living to a hundred.

"What is more those who knock up a century will not be

merely existing, predicts Dr. Edward Bortz, former president of the American Medical Association. In the majority of cases they will retain their faculties and be free of pain.

"Dr. Bortz's views are expressed in an article in the current issue of *Science Horizons*, published by the U.S. Embassy in London. The article points out that attempts to find anyone who has died simply of old age have always failed.

"One illness or another has always been responsible for ending a life. But as research yields more and more methods of defying disease the chances of living longer continue to grow.

"Just how long people in general could continue to live unencumbered by disease is not known but it is thought that 135 years would not be an unrealistic figure.

"In Dr. Bortz's opinion the reason comparatively few modern people live to a hundred or thereabouts is because they are unwilling to take regular exercise, watch their diet, have sufficient rest and recreation, and avoid handicapping themselves with stimulants and tranquillisers."

Remember nobody grows old by just living a number of years, but by giving up enthusiasm, faith, ideals, and self-confidence. We all retain the love of wonder, whether six or sixty, each day should be another great adventure into the wonder and mysteries of life, there is much to see, so much to do, so many people to help along life's pathway that we cannot afford to live in doubt, fear, and despair.

Someone long ago wrote: "You are young as your faith, as old as your doubts, as young as your self-confidence, as old as your fear, as young as your hope, and as old as your despair."

CHAPTER SEVEN

Of Interest to Women

I would like to clear away some of the fallacy, based on super-stition, that a woman may expect to suffer much distress, accompanied in many cases by severe pain, during the monthly cycle; that childbirth inevitably is a lengthy agonizing process; and that the change of life (menopause) must of necessity be a process of severe mental and physical discomfort.

Let us first deal with that oft-diagnosed condition known as dysmenorrhea, which means in effect an abnormal or disturbed menstrual cycle. There are many forms listed and described in the medical textbook and the description given of faulty position of the *uterus* and the *fallopian tubes* are undoubtedly true in many cases, and this can, and does, cause obstructive and mechanical dysme-norrhea. But, after seeing many partial and equally a great many complete cures of these effects, together with many cases of pre-vious miscarriages, having normal full-time delivery made possible entirely by the correction of the mechanical, spinal, and pelvic misalignment or distortion, your doctor of chiropractice does not consider that women's disorders should be tolerated, unless a correction of an apparent mechanical cause has first failed to bring relief.

Faulty position of the uterus and fallopian tubes occur when muscle tonicity, which should retain these organs in normal position, has been partially or wholly upset by previous strain or tear, such as an abnormally severe confinement. We feel a more prevalent cause is production of an inflammation of the nerve roots, by a subluxation of lumbar vertebrae and subsequent lumbo-sacral misalignment which reduces vital nerve impulses to the pelvic organs. In addition we often find a pelvic distortion adding to the resultant distress.

We know that many women are born with a displaced pelvis,

and thus we have, anatomically, imperfect balance; but in most of these cases the organs contained there are usually as adaptive as the organs within the skeletal structure of the hunchback. But in all cases we must be certain of the existence of normal transmission of nerve energy from brain and spinal cord to the pelvic basin.

It can be seen, therefore, that in many cases pelvic, and spinal adjustments to vertebrae, the lumbar, and often to the lower dorsals, are necessary to restore tone to the muscles and organs within that pelvis.

After many years of research we have found that nerves radiating from as high as the 9th or 10th dorsal or thoracic segments of the spine can elicit the usual symptoms of a vertebral subluxation in many cases of menstrual disorders.

One finds diminished mobility, increased skin temperature, tenderness to the touch, and hyperaemia, following such subluxations, and adjustments made to correct these local symptoms can hardly fail to have a beneficial effect on the organs and parts directly controlled by these nerve centres.

Usually doctors of chiropractice do not attempt to diagnose a condition of pelvic disorder as such. It is sufficient for them to find the region of nerve root interference, and, by making the necessary spinal adjustments there, to correct the disorder.

Diagnosis is the medical doctors' prerogative.

The chiropractor's is a spinal analysis.

We must remember that the effect of spinal adjustments on the nerves and blood vessels supplying the pelvic organs have a marked influence in producing healthy muscle tonicity, thereby permitting these organs to function perfectly. When there exists a diminished nerve impulse to one or any of the pelvic organs through pressure interference, either directly within the intervertebral foramina, upon the nerve roots, or indirectly through a general reduction of bodily nerve supply from the spinal canal due to vertebral bodies being out of juxtaposition with each other, especially in the Occipital, Atlanto-Axial region (the upper neck region).

The first vertebrae (the Atlas) when in malposition reduces the size of the Foramen Magnum (the opening through which the spinal cord passes to connect with the brain) and there exists compression of the surrounding tissues of the spinal cord. This can produce headaches, blackouts, sometimes a mild form of epilepsy, and, almost always, a diminishing of nerve energy normally conveyed to the body through the spinal cord and its network of nerves emitting from it.

We now have, as a result of this diminishing nerve activity, a general lowering of vitality and function, and the female pelvis is no exception to this.

As x-ray examination will prove, if the bony structures are in any way distorted, the pelvic organs are bound to be compressed in a similar way, if involved. Likewise if bony distortion occurs in the thorax (chest) the heart and lungs will be forced to one side or the other or become, as we say, adaptive.

When such bodily distortions are congenital (existing at birth) the imbalance of distortion is fixed and adaption more satisfactory, as with the hunchback, and no attempt should be made to bring about a correction that would conform to what we consider a normal pattern.

If, however, osseous (bony) structures are not permanently fixed in a distorted position, adaptation will be incomplete, because the adaptive measures which the body utilizes have to operate against a movable or variable force. We thus have strain, stress, wear, and tear, on surrounding tissue. Spinal and pelvic adjustments are then indicated, and will produce excellent results, very rewarding to the patient and operator alike.

It is thought by many laymen, and some doctors of medicine, that the degree of movement in the sacro-iliac articulation is either non-existent, or so limited, that it could not possibly affect the organs and parts contained within the pelvic basin. While we are aware that movement is seldom evident in the over-sixties, as we go down the scale towards the forties, thirties, to the adolescents, we find a continually increasing amount of movement within the articulation. As any joint through strain or malposition is incapable of full movement, so we find in the sacro-iliac joint movement of an eccentric (irregular) manner.

Being one of the main foundations of bodily balance, it is essential to maintain the pelvic articulations in as normal a position as possible, as it has to contend with all the jars, strains, and sometimes restricted powers of balanced locomotion in man's effort to maintain an erect position.

It is quite usual during a consultation with women complaining
of distress in the pelvic region accompanied by headaches,
irritability, depression, and often hysteria, for them to state
quite definitely that they were perfectly fit before they had their
first, and in some cases, their last child. Whilst we are aware that
such is a possibility, and are familiar with the adjustments which
the body makes to meet the ever changing weight and position
of a child before delivery, and in some cases by an abnormally
severe labour, we must not lose sight of the fact that a great
number of these women had low spine misalignments, a twisted
pelvis, or sacro-iliac tilt, long before the baby was conceived.

It follows that the abnormal distribution of weight during the
pre-natal period had merely increased the distortion and discomfort, sometimes producing an almost permanent disability, which
could have been prevented.

After thirty years of practice I feel confident that if correction
of spine and pelvic displacements had been made (preferably
before conception) and again during the immediate post-natal
period, we could have produced a notable reduction in the number
of women complaining of low back pain and, frequently, prolapse of the uterus in many instances. The prolapse was due to
reduction of nerve distribution and muscle tone, through compression of nerve roots which, in many cases, follows spinal
displacements in the lumbar and pelvic area of the body.

Some few years ago a bride of three and a half months arrived
at my surgery with a cheque, made out in the form of a wedding
present, which the giver had stipulated was to be used to obtain
spinal and pelvic x-rays. This was attached to a guarantee that
the party would pay for any necessary spinal manipulations should
these prove necessary.

I thought afterwards, what a wonderful way of expressing their
best wishes to the bride, preventing needless discomfort and pain,
making it possible to ensure the correction of spinal and pelvic
imbalance before the serious business of child-bearing.

Much of the irritability, depression, and panic hysteria that
accompanies the approach to the Climacteric, or change of
life, can be laid at the door of pelvic discomfort and low back
pain.

These could have been avoided had it been possible to have

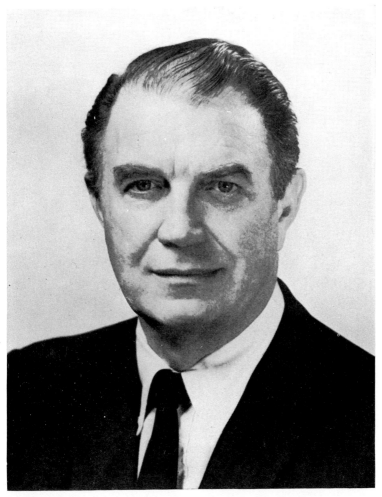

3. David D. Palmer, D.C., Ph.C., President, The Palmer College of Chiropractic, since 1961.

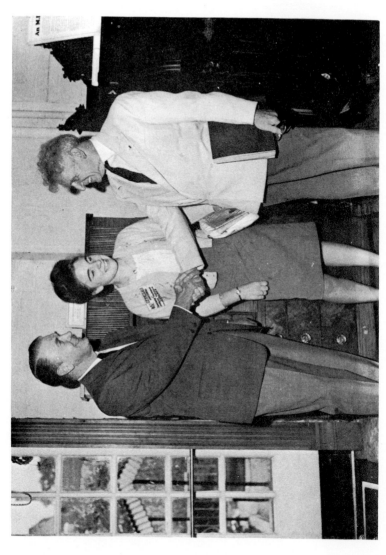

4. Dr. David D. Palmer, President of Palmer College, welcoming the author (and his daughter Heather) to

made available the services of the doctor of chiropractice in conjunction with the expert advice of the gynaecologist.

The menopause should be a natural process, gently swinging from one stage to another. It should not be accompanied by explosions of temper, irritability, long moods of depression, brain storms, or insanity. This may be only a physiological state.

Pain and distress, as in many other physical disabilities, can and often do have mental repercussions, so eliminate the cause of your backaches if you wish to retain your normal healthy attitude to life during this period of change.

With the elimination of spinal and pelvic imbalance by corrective chiropractic adjustments that may have had a direct bearing on women's reproductive life, it would be wise to turn our thoughts and action to some of the conditions that could occur in the event of a pregnancy.

All possible precautions should be taken to prevent the loss of the child before, during, and after the birth process. There are still too many cases of infant mortality, a great number of which could be avoided with a little more forethought and planning, and full co-operation with your family doctor.

For example, should the x-ray examination for low spine, sacral, and pelvic misalignments, reveal an exceptionally narrow pelvis, or on examination, a malposition of the baby, or an exceptionally large baby, you should request hospital admission for the birth. This will ensure that preventative and emergency facilities are available if required, because any one or combination of the above mentioned abnormal conditions may result in brain injuries, from which the death of the child could result if the confinement occurred elsewhere with the attendant risk of delay in receiving professional attention.

Do not take drugs of any kind unless with the consent, or preferably, the prescription of the doctor whom you are expecting to attend you at the confinement. There are still a great number of deaths caused by congenital malformations, some known, but many unknown, therefore do not take unnecessary risks with drugs. Remember the Thalidomide disaster. What greater proof of the unpredictable cause of disfigurement (or merciful death) caused by the little known permanent effect of drugs could you wish for?

Premature births carry a high incidence of infant mortality, and while haemorrhage and "maternal high blood pressure" are in the high category of possible causes, let us not forget that it has been established that women who smoke are twice as liable to have premature births as non-smokers. It is wise to give up smoking some months before conception "as is possible with planned families". Not only will you be giving up a health destroying habit, but you will be assuring a healthy baby.

Women having twins, women smokers, unmarried mothers, the very young mother, or the over-forties, have the highest incidence of low birth weight babies.

In this present age, in spite of appearing rather old-fashioned, I must add a possible additional preventative to curtail infant mortality amongst those "born live". That is for the mother to breast feed her baby for at least the first three or four weeks of its life unless otherwise directed by her doctor.

Babies found dead in their cots and bed are still far too numerous, and apart from the usual precautions taken against infection, the use of hard pillows, or none at all, suffocation still takes its toll; the possibility of regurgitation of cow's milk or other substitutes due to hypersensitivity must be seriously considered as an additional hazard in what are commonly known as "cot deaths".

Breast feeding after a few weeks may be discontinued if so desired, or continued if you wish. At any rate, see that your doctor is consulted about this, and his advice followed. You may thereby save yourself a lot of heartache, or even prevent a subsequent nervous breakdown.

CHAPTER EIGHT

Spinal Balance and its effect on the health and well-being of us all

The basis for the development of spinal balance and spinal hygiene condensed here are the findings of Leo J. Steinbach, D.C., of the faculty of the Universal Chiropractic College (now affiliated with the Lincoln Chiropractic College) and were compiled between 1920 and 1930, and it is reasonable to suppose that the percentages shown have increased due to the neglect of the spine, lowering muscle tonicity associated with the demands of modern civilization, and the hazards associated with mechanization.

The subjects studied in the research include an almost equal distribution of both sexes. Practically every trade, occupation, and profession is represented. Among 10,000 adult subjects studied for balance of the spine and variations from the normal contours of the body, the following deviations were found:

40% of all subjects showed unequal length of the lower extremities (differences of less than $\frac{1}{4}$ inch were not recorded.)
65% of all subjects showed unequal height of the shoulders.
60% of all subjects showed faulty neck or head carriage.
53% of all subjects showed deviations from the normal depth and/or length of antero-posterior curves of the spine.
77% of all subjects showed rotations in various parts of the spinal column.
10% of all subjects showed reasonably normal balance of the spine and body symmetry.

The plan for examination of the spinal column for defects of balance as herein outlined and the suggestions and recommendations for the listing and adjusting of vertebrae proceed from prolonged and careful efforts to discover the most effective method of reducing spinal subluxations.

It is not the purpose of this chapter to convey the impression that a perfect system of chiropractic examination and adjusting has been found.

It is offered rather as an improvement upon the original methods and as a plan that is completely in accord with the principle of vertebral adjustments as set forth in the literature of chiropractice and as laid down in the laws governing the chiropractic system of practice.

The results obtained through twenty-five years of progressive clinical work amply confirm the merit of the system. Problem cases have become fewer and the correction more lasting.

The utilization of the foregoing findings has led the workers of the research to look with favour upon the idea of employing corrective exercises to supplement the spinal adjustment. The restoration of tone and balance to the muscles and ligaments that support the spine adds value to the chiropractic adjustment and serves the good purpose of permitting the patient to share the responsibility of his case.

Examination of the spine for defects of antero-posterior balance:

NORMAL ANTERO-POSTERIOR BALANCE

The spinal column is flexible, and therefore, has a certain capacity to change according to the requirements of habits or occupations. It is also subject to the law of heredity, which means that it does not always have an original capacity to be mechanically perfect.

Like the face and other parts of the body, it does carry some of the distinctions of the family tree. However, in the main, the structure of the bones, cartilages, and supporting ligaments have sufficient similarity in the human family to describe the type of spinal column that conforms best to the requirements of life if the human body is to have the greatest capacity for action in the "vertical position".

1. Primarily, the spinal column is intended to furnish protection for the spinal cord and its nerve branches.
2. It is also intended to act as a weight-bearing structure.
3. It serves the purpose of a central axis for body movements.

4. It is a balance mechanism, striving always to keep body weight in a state of mechanical equilibrium with the least possible expenditure of nerve energy and muscular effort.

5. It is a compensating mechanism in that it adjusts and changes itself according to the demands or conditions found in other portions of the weight-bearing structures (lower extremities, pelvis, and ribs).

6. Finally, it is a shock absorber for the body by reason of its cartilages, curves, and flexibility. The shock-absorbing qualities of the spine, as an important phase of spinal functions, may be seriously impaired by defects of antero-posterior balance. An abnormal spinal curve that requires the weight of the body to be borne by only a part of the intervertebral disc causes thinning of the disc in that aspect and lowers the shock-absorbing powers of the spine.

In order to serve its six functions most effectively, the spinal column must have a certain antero-posterior balance, which should conform closely to the following description:

The 24 movable bones and the 23 intervening cartilages, some 28 inches in length for the average adult spine, must contain three curves:

Two curves in the anterior direction, cervical and lumbar.

One curve in the posterior direction, dorsal, or thoracic.

For normal weight balance in the spine, the single posterior curve should be 12 vertebrae long, and the two anterior curves (cervical and lumbar) should include 12 vertebrae. Thus, in the mechanically perfect spinal column, one half of the column should curve backward in one curve, and one half should curve forward in two curves. The sacrum, which is the keystone in the arch of the pelvis, is a relatively unchangeable section of the spinal column, although the angle of its upper surface or base helps to decide the depth and length of the lumbar curve. In the normal state it is intended to have a fixed position through articulation with the innominate bones.

For perfect anterior-posterior balance or posture, the three curves should merge smoothly with each other and should enjoy easy unions with the skull above and the sacrum below. In order to retain good capacity to sustain its six functions, the cervical, dorsal, and lumber curves of the spine should have a certain comparative depth. For the normal spinal column, the depth of the curves should vary somewhat according to the weight and in proportion to the height of the individual.

Normal antero-posterior balance combined with average weight and height provides the body with:

1. Good appearance.
2. Flexibility.
3. The maximum range of action.
4. The best possible adaptability to the pursuits of life.

With normal balance, the spine acts as an effective shock absorber, helping to make energy last longer. The natural object of chiropractic therapy and hygiene is to preserve the normal curves of the spine.

Figures 1 to 4 are examples of correct antero-posterior balance or posture.

Figure 1 illustrates graphically how body weight is distributed in relation to the central axis or gravity line; it also shows the system of levers that support this weight. Studying this figure carefully will induce a better understanding of how antero-posterior balance faults will change natural weight balance and produce undue strain to the muscles and ligaments.

Note principally:

1. The carriage of the head.
2. Chest carriage.
3. The position of the spine in relation to weight distribution of the body.
4. The depth of the anterior cervical and lumbar curves and the posterior dorsal curve as related to the gravity line.
5. The position of the sacrum.
6. The system of muscles, illustrated with dotted lines, demonstrating the balancing mechanism of levers that permit the upright position and also flexor and extensor movements of the body.
7. The axis by which weight is transmitted to the lower extremities.

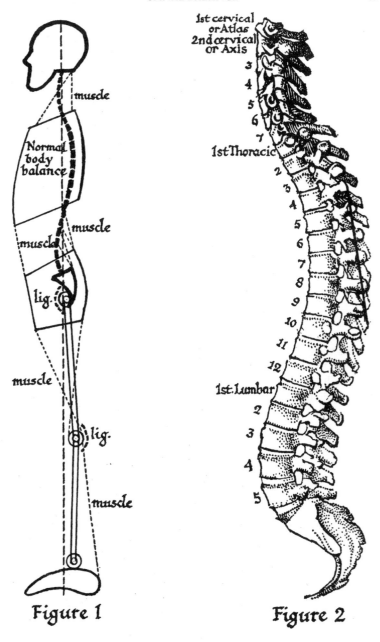

muscle

Normal
body
balance

muscle

muscle

lig.

muscle

lig.

muscle

Figure 1

1st cervical
or Atlas
2nd cervical
or Axis
3
4
5
6
7
1st Thoracic
2
3
4
5
6
7
8
9
10
11
12
1st Lumbar
2
3
4
5

Figure 2

8. The length of the curves of the spine, comparing one to another and the even or gradual blending of one curve into another. The least strain is recorded upon the muscles and ligaments when the spinal column has a reasonably exact length and depth to its several curves. The ability of the spine to withstand shock and physical strain is directly dependent upon a correctly curved spinal column.

Figure 2 is a lateral view of the normal vertebral column, as taken from *The Anatomy of the Human Body* by Gray. The following description of "The Vertebral Column as a Whole" subheading "Curves" is taken from Gray and should be studied carefully.

"Viewed laterally, the vertebral column presents several curves, which correspond to the different regions of the column, and are called cervical, thoracic, lumbar, and pelvis. The cervical curve, convex forward, begins at the apex of the odontoid process, and ends at the middle of the second thoracic vertebra; it is the least marked of all the curves.

"The thoracic curve, concave forward, begins at the middle of the second and ends at the middle of the twelfth thoracic vertebra. Its most prominent point behind corresponds to the spinous process of the seventh thoracic vertebra.

"The lumbar curve is more marked in the female than in the male; it begins at the middle of the last thoracic vertebra, and ends at the sacrovertebral angle. It is convex anteriorly, the convexity of the lower three vertebrae being much greater than that of the upper two. The pelvic curve begins at the sacrovertebral articulation, and ends at the point of the coccyx; its concavity is directed downward and forward. The thoracic and pelvic curves are termed primary curves, because they alone are present during foetal life.

"The cervical and lumbar curves are compensatory or secondary, and are developed after birth, the former when the child is able to hold up its head (at three or four months), and to sit upright (at nine months), the latter at twelve or eighteen months, when the child begins to walk. The vertebral column has also a slight lateral curvature, the convexity of which is directed towards the right side."

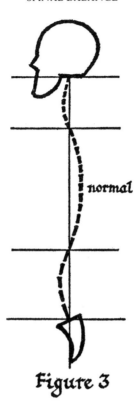

normal

Figure 3

Figure 3 is an illustration of the spinal column more simple in form than that of Figure 2.

Study it carefully and apply the facts as stated in the quotation from Gray's *Anatomy*. The terminology differs from that mentioned by Gray in that the cervical and lumbar curves will be called anterior curves, and the dorsal and pelvic curves will be called posterior curves.

Note particularly in Figure 3 the blending of the cervical and dorsal curves, with their union between the seventh cervical and first and second dorsal vertebrae; note also the blending of the dorsal and lumbar curves, the union between the two normally involving the twelfth dorsal and first lumber vertebrae.

All union points should be as merges, sharp unions or "breaks" are points of strain and may be classified as weakened areas where trouble is likely to develop.

Note also the apex points of each of the three curves; that of the cervical curve is rarely seen elsewhere than at the level of the fourth cervical. The dorsal curve has its apex point at the junction between the sixth and seventh dorsal vertebrae; and the lumbar curve presents its greatest anteriority at the level of the third lumbar vertebra. These values are all normals.

Figure 4 illustrates the normal spine projected into the body and the characteristic that normal or correct spinal values impart to the body outlines.

The curves of the spine have a certain length and depth; these values when preserved avoid the development of undue strain to the ligaments and muscles of the body and prevent harmful nerve irritations. The proper curving of the spine provides the body with good carriage and easy balance of weight. When associated with correct body balance, unnecessary expenditure of nervous and muscular energy is avoided, and the body is provided with the proper basis for good health.

EXAMINATION PROCEDURE FOR ANTERO-POSTERIOR BALANCE

Preparation.

For examination, the standing position is employed as the functional position of the body (Figure 5). In this position balance or posture, as well as all other physical characteristics, are displayed. Mechanical efficiency or inefficiency is best observed.

The subject should stand with the heels of the feet even and set 6 to 10 inches apart. Make sure that the feet are spaced as designated above. This stance places the feet directly below the heads of the femur bones and allows the subject to stand comfortably with the weight evenly distributed. The back should be well lighted and the examiner positioned slightly to one side and behind the subject in order to observe the character of the spinal curves.

The use of the plumb line is valuable, but its use will be curtailed as visual experience grows. This method of examination quickly trains the eye to appreciate variations of curves in different subjects.

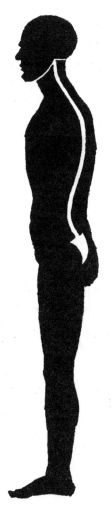
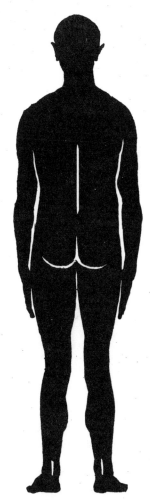

Figure 4 **Figure 5**

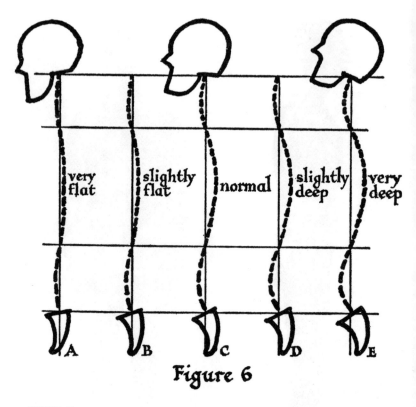

Figure 6

POINT 1

Estimate the depth of the cervical, dorsal, and lumbar curves. The spine may then be classified as one of the following types (See Figure 6):

A Definitely flat
B Moderately flat
C Normal depth
D Moderately deep
E Definitely deep

POINT 2

Observe the length of the dorsal and lumbar curves, noting the position of the apices and the smoothness of the dorso-lumbar junction. As designated under normal antero-posterior balance,

the dorsal curve demonstrates a normal length of twelve vertebrae; the anterior lumbar curve is five vertebrae long. The apices
of both curves should be at their normal level, respectively, the
junction between the sixth and seventh dorsals and the third
lumbar.

The union between the two curves should be accomplished
smoothly. Any deviation in the length of the curves should be
noted. The apex points of the two curves should be noted; abnormal positions are seen in which the dorsal apex may be as
high as the fourth dorsal (Figure 7) or as low as the tenth dorsal

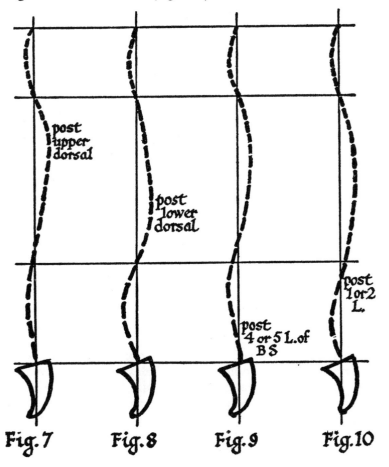

Fig. 7   Fig. 8   Fig. 9   Fig. 10

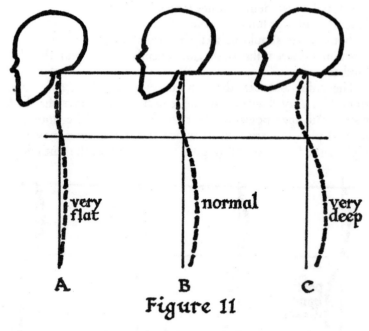

Figure 11

(Figure 8). In balance defects the lumabr apex may be as high as the first lumbar (Figure 9) or as low as the fourth or fifth lumbar (Figure 10).

In defects of balance the normally smooth union of the cervico-dorsal or dorso-lumbar junctions may be lost, the spine breaking sharply at or near the normal point of union (Figures 7 and 8). Sharp breaking unions of the cervico-dorsal and dorso-lumbar junctions are, in many instances, induced by posterior subluxations. When a posterior subluxation occurs near the normal point of union of spinal curves, it creates a sharp breaking union, with consequent strain at that point.

These types of defective antero-posterior balance were never observed by the public and have had little consideration even by the chiropractic profession. There are also frequent instances of change from the normal position of the apex point of the dorsal and lumbar curves due to posterior subluxation of vertebrae. When a posterior subluxation occurs near the normal apex of a curve, it invariably becomes the apex point of the curve.

These sharp-breaking unions are a point of strain in the spine; they impair both spinal shock-absorbing properties in that area and render the region of the spine affected susceptible to subluxation or further subluxation through shock. They lessen the general efficiency of the spine.

POINT 3

Observe head carriage from the side in order to estimate the depth of the cervical curve. In Figure 11 note the positions of the head in relation to the scomparative depth of the cervical curves.

In A (a very flat spine) the head is tilted forward, chin tucked into the neck. This type of posture believed by many to be correct balance is not. The flatness of the cervical curve diminishes its shock-absorbing power and creates strain in the muscles and ligaments of the neck.

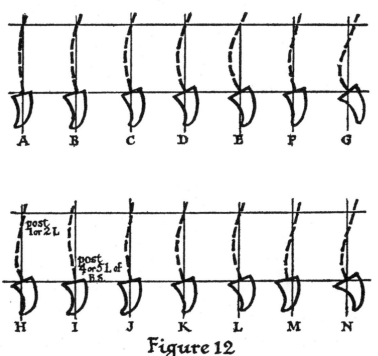

Figure 12

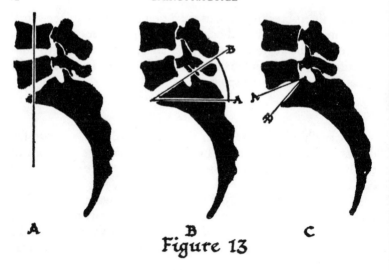

A   B   C

Figure 13

B presents normalcy of cervical curving, permitting the greatest efficiency of muscular action, good shock-absorbing qualities, and easy balance, of the weight of the head. The head, correctly carried, improves appearance, facilitates normal use of the eyes, speaking, and breathing. Make note of any deviations.

In C (a definitely deep spine) the deepness of the cervical curve causes the chin to be elevated and the head to be tipped backward.

POINT 4

Observe the carriage of the pelvis. Study the illustrations in Figure 12; note the variations in the relative position of the sacrum. Lateral x-ray films show graphically the position of the sacrum in relation to the position that the centre of gravity maintains; shifts in the antero-posterior balance of the lumbar spine and pelvic region are also readily detected.

The following values may be used when examining the lateral lumbar and pelvic x-ray film made in the standing position:

Centre of Gravity—a perpendicular dropped through the middle of the body of the third lumbar vertebra should pass through the anterior one fourth of the sacral base if weight bearing is normal (Figure 13a).

Lumbo-Sacral Angle—degree of anterior inclination of the sacral base from the horizontal—illustrated in Figure 13b, varies between 19 and 72 degrees, with an average of 37 degrees. (These figures are based upon 4,000 symptomless cases studied.) Line A is horizontal to the bottom of the film and intersects line B drawn through the base of the sacrum.

The Mobility of the Lumbo-Sacral Angle (measured in degrees) is determined by comparing the lumbo-sacral angle of a film made in the horizontal position with that made in the vertical position. The normal range of variation for the angle is 10 degrees greater in the vertical than in the horizontal position. The lumbo-sacral angle value greater or less than the normal 10 degree increase when in the vertical position generally presents symptoms; e.g. when several degrees less than 10 in the vertical position film are present, there is some compensatory muscular effort being made by the subject to maintain or open the intervertebral foramina: when the difference is greater than 10 degrees, the back, particularly the lumbo-sacral area, and all of its muscular and ligamentous ramifications is "weakened" or "unstable". (This conclusion is based upon 4,000 symptomless cases studied.)

The Facet Syndrome—when lines drawn through the inferior surface of the fifth lumbar vertebral body (line A) and through the base of the sacrum (line B) bisect anterior to the posterior neural arch, what is known as the Facet Syndrome is presented. The weight of the body is transferred from the lumbar vertebral bodies to the facets or articulating surfaces of the lumbar vertebrae. This may encroach upon the intervertebral foramina of the fourth and fifth lumbar nerves and may also cause spinous irritation of the lumbar vertebrae (Figure 13c).

Since it is not always practical, and somewhat costly, to x-ray the lumbar spine and pelvis laterally to determine the position of the sacrum in antero-posterior balance examinations, the visual powers must be cultivated in order to appreciate the position of the sacrum, the pelvis in general, and the lumbar spine.

As a general rule, the fifth lumbar and, to a somewhat lesser extent, the rest of the lumbar spine, will follow the position of the sacrum. The placement of the sacrum may be readily analysed both visually and by palpation. The plumb line may be of help in developing the visual powers. If the buttocks and the sacral apex

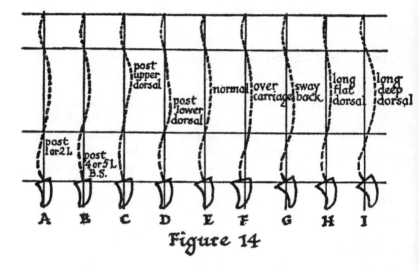

post
upper
dorsal

post
lower
dorsal

normal

over
carriage

sway
back

long
flat
dorsal

long
deep
dorsal

post
1 or 2 L

post
4 or 5 L
B.S.

A B C D E F G H I

Figure 14

are prominent, it naturally follows that the lumbo-sacral angle will be increased. Lumbar spinal curving is likely to be deep, there is a possibility of the facet syndrome being present, and the gravity line may pass the level of the sacrum anterior to the sacral base. Faulty pelvic and lumber balance of this type is most aptly illustrated as a "sway back" or a "long, deep dorsal curve" (Figure 14g and i, respectively). The long, deep dorsal curve is the classic example. It is a postural type indicating a weakened muscular system and may be associated with overweight and a pendulous abdomen.

Conversely, when the buttocks are not prominent and the sacral base, rather than the sacral apex, is especially noticeable, the lumbar curve is usually on the flat side. The pelvis is carried habitually too far forward, the gravity line passing through the sacrum in its posterior aspect. This condition is known as "over carriage" (Figure 14f). Walking becomes more difficult due to the strain of balancing the body in the erect position, the strain being transferred to the feet and legs. Corrective exercises to improve muscular tone in the "over carriage" postural type are essential.

POINT 5

Consider the advisability of making posterior listings in various sections of the spine.

Be governed by the following rules and suggestions:

1. Avoid posterior listings in flat dorsal and in deep lumbar curves.
2. Give favourable consideration to posterior vertebrae in deep dorsal curves and in flat lumbar and cervical curves.
3. Avoid posterior listings of the sixth or seventh dorsals when the dorsal apex is too high or too low. Give preference to vertebrae at abnormal apex.
4. Avoid the third lumbar as a posterior listing when the lumbar apex is too high or too low. When too high, give preference to the fourth or fifth lumbar or the base of the sacrum. When the apex is too low, give preference to posterior listing of upper lumbars.

SUMMARY

In the light of the observations made and notes taken under POINTS 2 to 5, the antero-posterior balance faults may be reclassified. Reconsider the back as explained under POINT 1. If the cause of a "slightly flat" spine (Figure 6b) is found to be the result of a posterior fourth or fifth lumbar vertebra or a posterior base of the sacrum, the "spinal type" then may be reclassified as to cause (as in Figure 14b). A listing may then be made with the choice of the fourth or fifth lumbar or base of the sacrum as posterior. Coupled with hygienic care and possible corrective exercise, the prognosis of the condition will be much improved.

If the "spinal type" is as in Figure 6e, the possible cause may be a posterior upper dorsal subluxation (Figure 14c). A long flat dorsal curve (Figure 14h) may be the result of a posterior lower dorsal or upper lumbar subluxation (Figure 14a and d).

It is generally well to look for a posterior subluxation where there exists a sharp-breaking union between curves or when a curve is too long.

CHAPTER NINE

The Spinal Adjustment, its action and effects

I think there is no more thrilling drama in history than that of sickness and its adjustment. There has been no one thing in the history of man that has done more to hold man down and make a prisoner out of him, than sickness, and there is no one thing that has done more to make criminals out of people, than the subluxation and its influence upon the human race. So we will call this chapter "The Spinal Adjustment, its action and effects".

Let us first state that an adjustment given skilfully with speed and a torque-like movement is the thrust made by the hands of your doctor of chiropractice in the correct direction, with sufficient toggle to create a movement of a misaligned, or subluxated vertebra, with sufficient precision to reduce cleavage surrounding such a vertebra without resultant pain.

For those who have no bent towards engineering or movements sometimes connected with it, let us describe the toggle movement and simplify it as follows:

If you held a 2 in nail on to a piece of wood and placed a 7 lb hammer on its head, and pressed it hard with all your weight, you would not indent the wood more than about $\frac{1}{8}$ in, but, if you replaced the 7 lb hammer with one of say 8 oz total weight, lifted it into the air, and struck a blow on to the top of a nail you would, without striking a severe blow, produce an indentation into the wood of at least $\frac{1}{4}$ in. Again, if using the same light hammer, you wiggle the nail and hit it while in motion you would more than double the indentation depth made by the nail because you have reduced the repellent action of the surrounding wood fibre round your nail point, or as we say, reduced cleavage.

Just as is in the question of disease and the subluxation that is the cause of the dis-ease, you have got to do more than merely study the effect itself, which is the dis-ease.

To understand it thoroughly you must study the *cause* of much *disease*; the *subluxation*; the *specific cause*. In order to understand this you have to understand the general nature of what causes subluxations in order to know what to do to adjust them.

In all of nature there are two forces at work, the centripetal and the centrifugal, the hub and the rim, the inside and the outside, the invasion and the resistance. There is no movement of any matter that is not moved upon by energy, and any matter that is designed to be moved upon by energy, offers resistance to being moved. So we find two forces at work, that from the hub to the rim, and that from the rim to the hub, the centripetal force resisting the centrifugal, the centrifugal resisting the centripetal, the invasion force trying to get in, the resistance force trying to keep it out.

What is force? It is that abstract energy, which even as an abstract, is still abstract energy, but does not become released by movement as an energy until it attempts to remove matter. There would be no movement of matter if it were not that matter refused to be resisted by its movement.

The nearest example we have to that principle of physics is that there is electricity in the atmosphere. We have energy here; the energy cannot be seen or felt nor sensed by any human sense. When this energy is condensed, concentrated, boiled down into an essence, and stored away into a battery, then released into some other form of matter such as gunpowder, it can do a tremendous amount of damage when the gunpowder resists its action. If the energy in a room could be condensed into a battery, and released into gunpowder it would do that same thing, because as it met with resistance from the energy contained within the gunpowder, one trying to get in and the other trying to keep it out, the clash between the two would blow a town to pieces.

There is enough electricity in the air within any room to light a globe, but it will never do so unless through a generator meeting with resistance in transmission. That resistance produces work, and work produces heat, and heat produces *white heat* which produces white light.

Electricity of itself does not produce light, never has and never will. Electricity moves matter, thus making energy in action. Energy makes work, makes the motor work, and when the motor works, the motor gets hot, and when it gets hot it gets white, and when it gets white, it generates a by-product, light. Light is a by-product of a white colour, and a white colour is a by-product of heat. Heat is a by-product of work; work is a by-product of resistance, and resistance is a by-product of an invasion; invasion is a by-product of transmission.

Many times Thomas A. Edison was asked what electricity was. His reply invariably was the same: "I do not know. Why do you ask? Hundreds of others have asked me the same question."

"But, Mr Edison, when we push the button on the wall what do we do?"

"Nothing."

"But," people said, "we get light in the globe in the ceiling."

"That is right," he said, "when we push the button we get the light from the ceiling."

"And why do we get a light at a point distant from the button?"

Thomas Edison said, "We would not have light if we did not push the button."

"When I push the button I do something that makes the light possible at the other end of the wire?"

"Again," Thomas Edison said, "you do not."

"What is electricity?"

"Again," he said, "I don't know."

"Well, how does the electricity get from the button to the globe or to the ceiling? Does it go over the wire or through the wire?"

He said, "I think it goes through the wire, but I don't know."

Marconi was asked, "Does electricity go through the wire or over the wire?" He said, "Neither in my opinion, neither way." To illustrate he said, "Suppose you laid down a pile of balls in a line, and you were to tap the one on the end, the other one on the other end rolls off and all the other balls between stand still; a billiard player will tell you that. How they move, that is atomic pressure. You transfer the atomic pressure of the first ball to the second, the second to the third, and finally by the atomic pressure passing along, from ball to ball, it gets to the last one and the last one rolls off."

"Now," Marconi said, "nothing went from ball to ball except pressure, and pressure is energy, and so when it comes to the study of energy or forces at work we have one of the most complex studies there is."

In a similar way, a chiropractic adjustment is a concussion of force upon a resistant object, namely, the spinal vertebra.

Our main concern at the moment is with the working principle, that there are two forces always at work. For instance light, colour, sound, taste, acid, alkalines, are all forces. Anything which comes to your body and gets in is an energy getting in, whether it be obvious or not. The only difference between the low note on the piano and the high, is the difference between black and white, or any of the shades between. The only difference between bitter and sweet, between harsh and pleasant, is the quantity of energy that is trying to invade you.

Now forces are constantly bombarding your body. They might bombard it as light coming into the eye, or they might bombard it in the form of noise coming into your ear. They might bombard it in the form of a taste coming into your food, or they might bombard it in the form of a sensation. You may note the things which you feel with your hands or your skin. Yet it is an invasionary force. Your body in return is resisting this invasion. Primarily we are concerned that you recognize the simple principle that there are two forces at work, one on the outside trying to get in, and the other inside trying to keep it out.

Now the difference between these two principles, and the interpretation placed upon them, is, that within us we have an innate intelligence which receives the impression at the surface, the energy trying to get in is taken up to the seat of resistance and the innate intelligence may state: "You are an energy I need; I want you; I welcome you to come in." It also says to other forces, "You are dangerous; you are injurious; you are harmful; I do not want you; keep out; get out", and if the force still tries to get in, innate tries to keep it out. The two forces are in conflict. Whether a force is a welcome force or an injurious one, is a question of the interpretation placed upon it by innate intelligence, and its successful repulse, if injurious, depends upon the expression of the forces of innate intelligence at the point of invasion. The outside force as it meets with resistance may do damage. If it meets with a welcome reception it can do no damage.

Now let us put it into figures or percentages to illustrate one point more clearly. Over twenty-five years ago B. J. Palmer gave a lecture to many of us in which he endeavoured to drive into our minds an appreciation of body resistance and reception. I remembered it and quote from my notes: "If the invasionary force is 100% and if the resistance force is 100% then we have the old, old problem of physics, because if an irresistible force meets an immovable object, neither will move the other. It is like putting two engines nose to nose on the same track. One has exactly the same power as the other. When we turn on the steam of both engines, they will both stand still; neither one will move the other, but if one engine has but the advantage of one horse-power over the other it will push it back.

"Now if the invasionary force is 105% and the resistance is 100% you have 5% of invasion to overcome resistance, and harm is going to result. Or if the invasionary force is 100% and the resistance force is 85% we are going to have 15% damage, and this is going to *do* damage. What do I mean by damage? I mean by that, we can have fractures, dislocations, subluxation and misalignments so far as it affects osseous structural framework. Beyond that I am not concerned, because I, as a chiropractor, if it produces a prolapse of a viscera, or the tearing and rending of the skin, or the breaking of a bone, have nothing to do with that. That is in the field of surgery and not in my province. I am concerned with the invasionary force so far as it disarranges the osseous structure, or the framework as it applies to the articulations of the body.

"Now when two forces are in conflict, if the invasionary force is greater than the resistance, harm will be the result, but if the invasionary force is 50% and the resistance 100% or 85% or anything over 50%, no harm will occur.

"We have four degrees of possible injury to osseous structure which are, *fractures, dislocations, subluxations* and *misalignments*. A fracture is of greatest invasionary value with the least resistance. A dislocation is less than a fracture, and has less than a fracture value and more than a fracture value in resistance. A subluxation is less than a dislocation value, and more than the resistance of a dislocation value.

"In other words, let us put it his way. It takes more force to produce a fracture in any back-bone, than it does a dislocation.

It takes more invasionary value in quantity of force to produce a dislocation, than it does a subluxation. It takes more force to produce a subluxation, than it does a misalignment, and the reverse of these is true of the invasionary force and the resistant force.

"Now in this structural framework we are taught, as a matter of osteology, that our head sits on something and that our arms hang off of something, that our legs hang off of something. What is it? The back-bone. The back-bone is the centre to which and from which, all energies radiate in or out. It is obvious that the word back-bone is something more than merely a word. It means more than merely an assemblage of individual back-bones.

"The back-bone is just what it theoretically implies: that all forces concentrate to it, and all forces radiate from it. Any force approaching your body will concentrate and strike at that back-bone, just the same as when you hurl a rock into a pool of water, it will send out waves which eventually reach a bank and there at the bank it will do damage, or not do damage, according to its invasionary force meeting with resistance. Now all meeting of opposing forces radiate waves, which hit the back-bone, and from the back-bone we resist that wave that comes towards it.

"All these vertebrae are interlaterally locked. Coming down through the centuries the spinal column has been definitely locked to prevent any damage to it. As I hypothetically said, however, I do not believe innate has quite finished the job, and two of the vertebrae are still without her inter-articulatory locks, to prevent them being subluxated, so that any force approaching this body anywhere can, and eventually does, radiate to that back-bone and they will do no harm except at the place where harm can be done, which is at the vertebra where it is not locked, which means the occipital, atlas and axis articulation. *At that point we can have a subluxation.*

"We can have a fracture anywhere else; we can have dislocations anywhere else, but we can only have subluxations where there are no inter-articulatory locks. We can have misalignments anywhere in the back-bone, or anywhere else in the body, but we can only have a subluxation at a point where there are none of these inter-articulatory locks, that is at *occiput, atlas* and *axis*.

"Now where two forces clash as a result of which they twist

and distort, and wrench a vertebra out of its natural position, as a result there is a *subluxation*.

"Light has its range from black to white just as heat has its range from severe cold in the winter to extreme heat in the summer, or just as there is a range in the voice of the female or the male, from the lesser number of vibrations per second of the vocal chords to the higher number of vibrations. It is this difference in the range of vibrations per second, between the female voice and the male voice, that constitutes the difference between the basso profundo of the male, and the high soprano of the female.

"We have a different range of motion in a fracture, and a still greater difference in a dislocation, or in a misalignment. Subluxations also have a range of motion, what I call the hub or the rim of the roof of the subluxation within its range.

"Having proved that a concussion of forces causes a subluxation, wherein the invasionary force was greater than the resistance, because of the peculiar twisting nature of it, it was like a torque and was torqued into a subluxation, and now it will stay; but even as it will stay it will rise and fall in its range of motion from minute to minute, hour to hour, and day to day.

"Your doctor of chiropractice must learn that to adjust a subluxation one must reverse the working principle that caused the subluxation, and until he learns that he is not getting anywhere (for unless he does learn that the concussion of force that he seeks to apply to correct the subluxation, must be a reversal), his concussion may but add its effect to the prior concussion that produced the subluxation. He must also learn that his adjustment is an invasionary force to what now exists there, and the body of the patient is going to offer resistance, and that now there is going to be a clash of conflict—the concussion of the two forces. The force that he is going to introduce, and the force with which the body is going to resist—after all it is a state of invasion and resistance—the greater resistance I have to attack my invasion, the more and greater invasion I would have to attack and break down the resistance. If I had no resistance then it does not take much invasionary force to get in. If I can lower his resistance the less invasionary force I have to break down the resistance, which is obvious.

"*This is one reason why I do all in my power to get the patient to relax before we administer the adjustment.* We want to reduce the resistance to the invasionary force that we are to apply and to do that one must use every trick that one can, to overcome the resistance on the part of the patient.

"Now there are many ways in which to overcome the patient's resistance, and, also there are many ways to increase his resistance to your adjustment. The doctor of chiropractice who carefully analyses his x-ray films, determines what has to be adjusted, and confidently places his hands upon the patient's spine, and upon obtaining a relaxing effect by calm assurance, it is possible to make an adjustment to a subluxation, *without any pain.*

"The new doctor in many cases, hesitates and shows his inability to assess the patient's resistance, by constant wiggling, friction, movement of hands while he is getting into position to correct this subluxation. This alone increases body resistance to adjustment of a subluxation, and the result can be a mildly painful movement which tends to create a form of future resistance to any further adjustments that are to be made. The patient likewise can give great assistance to the doctor by relaxing early and, if possible, taking his mind off the actual forthcoming movement of the vertebrae. It requires little invasionary force to overcome resistance from a relaxed patient, and it likewise requires little adjustic force to correct the subluxated vertebrae. A patient who is thoroughly relaxed at the moment that the invasionary forces get in (innate being relaxed), comes right back and concentrates everything. She is not (in resistance), and then when she comes back at me with that little vertebrae it wiggles around in there with that recoil action, and *innate* puts it where it belongs.

"*Your doctor of chiropractice does not do this; Innate does it.* It is innate that could not prevent the subluxation, and it is *innate that makes the adjustment,* not your doctor. I never gave an adjustment in my life, and never will, but the innate in the patient is what is making the adjustment, and by getting relaxation my invasionary force gets in, and by having them relaxed innate can now react upon my invasion and set that vertebrae back, and set it exactly where it belongs. *Innate can do that—I cannot.* I do not know where that line is, innate does. I make innate do my work for me.

"A skilfully applied chiropractic adjustment produces chemical changes in addition to producing mobility, then moves and thrusts stimulate reflexes—that is they tend to increase the flow of arterial blood through a given part, to ease the congestion of venous blood and lymph. But they do more than that. *Blood sugar is a vital constituent of adrenalin* and another vital fluid called *sympathin*. The release of these vital fluids stimulates the activity of body hormones which are the life givers and healing agents.

"The specific thrust from the chiropractor will touch the self-starter and set in motion the vast machinery housed in the living framework of that wonderful body of yours."

CHAPTER TEN

Medical Opposition and Investigations, Translation from German M.D's Observations, Chiropractic Philosophy

In spite of the wealth of references from medical literature pointing to the efficacy of chiropractic procedure, organized medicine continues to oppose chiropractice progress. Although individual medical practitioners in certain instances show signs of co-operating, the profession generally continues its policy of rejection. This works a hardship on patients seeking health care and creates difficulty for the members of our profession. We feel the basic reason to this opposition is in error, and is not in the public interest.

Orthodox medicine has frequently opposed valuable new procedures in the field of health, and has even ridiculed some of its own famous researchers as fools and frauds.

History is repeating itself, and we refer to statements made at the Convention of the Canadian Medical Association in Banff in July 1960 by Dr. W. B. Parsons of Red Deer, Alberta. Dr. Parsons was frank in his address, and spoke out strongly in favour of the methods used by chiropractors. The principal points covered in his talk were as follows:

Rejection of Manipulative Therapy was sometimes emotional, and reminded him of the opposition to Lister, Pasteur and Hunter. He said the medical profession is wrongly critical of the manipulation of backs. He said that manipulative claims had been too extravagant, but that some of the blame for this state of affairs lies with the medical profession due to its lack of understanding of, or failure to recognize, certain types of back pain. He also advised that physicians should not condemn doctors of chiropractice for their mistakes, for we cannot hide the fact that their

successes are our failures. Dr Parson's reasons for studying
chiropractice are clearly outlined in an article which he prepared
in conjunction with D. J. A. Cumming, M.D., and which was
published in the Canadian Medical Association *Journal*, 15th July
1958, Volume 79, page 103, Appendix I.

Dr. Parsons explains the reason that he took up manipulation
was an interest in backache with the early discovery that many
patients who fail to respond to routine medical treatment went
to a manipulator and received immediate benefit. This discovery
was followed by the acceptance of the classic advice "*If you can't
whip 'em, join 'em*" at least to the extent of borrowing their
technique.

The Canadian Medical Association *Journal*, 1st April 1959,
Vol. 78, Appendix 3, provides a report which was translated
from German on chiropractice methods. This report is an outcome of the intensive investigation into chiropractice which has
taken place in Germany in the last few years, and which is
referred to in more detail in the book *Medicine and Chiropractic*,
Exhibit 13. The report is entitled "*Pain Syndromes originating in
the Vertebral Column and their amenability to manipulative treatment*"
(the last two words of the title have been altered in the translation from "Chiropractic treatment" to read "Manipulative
treatment"). For an accurate translation see page 119 *Medicine and
Chiropractic*, Exhibit 13, under Supplemental references Leeman
R. A. The author refers to it as "Improvements in diagnosis and
Treatment of many painful conditions through an improved
awareness of the importance of spinal mechanics". He states that
chiropractice procedures permit the treatment of the cause of
certain conditions rather than the effect. He also supports the
five chiropractice principles. He states that subluxations are of
particular importance in regard to nerve root compression and
describes them as a locking of the joints. He explains that abolition
of such locking by chiropractic manœuvres would explain the
startling relief of pain from them in such cases.

The *investigation into chiropractic methods in Germany since World
War II*, represent the only scientific study conducted by the
medical profession on this subject. The results have been highly
favourable. One has merely to read the references at the bottom
of each page of *Medicine and Chiropractic* and the pages of

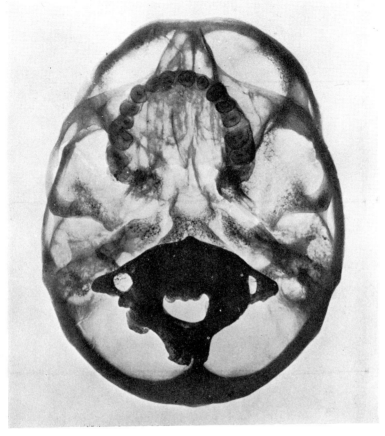

5. Photograph of the actual specimen after dissolution of all the osseous inorganic structure by the famous "Spalteholtz" process. Original specimen is permanently exhibited at The Palmer College of Chiropractic, Davenport, Iowa, U.S.A.

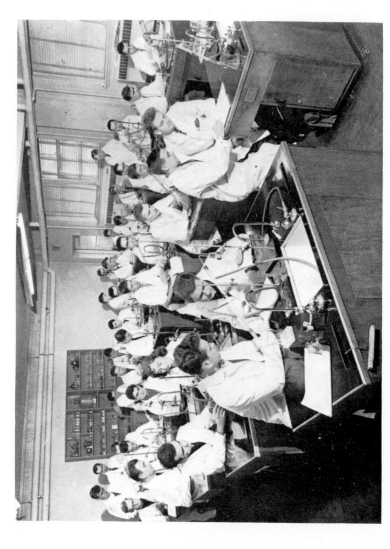

6. Students in a corner of the chemistry and physics laboratory, Canadian Memorial College, Toronto.

Supplementary References, pages 118, 119, 120, 121, to understand the scope and depth of study and the favourable outcome.

Medicine in North America commenced its ridicule of chiropractic practice almost as far back as 1895 without having seriously studied the subject. It is true that some early chiropractors made extravagant claims. It is also true that the outright denial of the scientific basis of sound chiropractice principle by medicine is equally wrong. It is our opinion that medical treatments being given for conditions which have been incorrectly diagnosed demonstrates the lack of understanding of the significance of referred pain from the joints of the spine as stated by J. Mennell, John McM. Mennell, W. V. Parsons, R. A. Leeman, J. E. Goldthwaite, Sidney Light and many others.

What is Chiropractice?

1. It is appropriate at this stage of our writings to quote the interpretation selected by the Canadian Chiropractic Association in their brief to the Royal Commission on Health Services before its Chairman, the Hon. Emmett Hall, Chief Justice of Saskatchewan, in 1961–62, which officially defines chiropractice as the philosophy, science and art of locating, correcting and adjusting the interference with nerve transmission and expression in the spinal column and other articulations without the use of drugs or surgery.

2. In addition, the chiropractice profession endorses the World Health Organization definition that health is a state of physical, mental and social well-being, and not merely the absence of disease and infirmity.

3. The science of chiropractic deals with the relationship between the articulations of the human body, especially the vertebral column, and the nervous system, and the role of these relationships in the restoration and maintenance of health.

4. The philosophy of chiropractice is based upon the premise that disease or abnormal function is frequently caused by interference with nerve transmission and expression, due to deviation from their normal position of the bony segments of the body, especially the vertebral column.

5. The practice of chiropractice consists of the location and correction of misalignments causing any interference with normal

nerve transmission and expression, for the restoration and maintenance of health without the use of drugs or surgery.

Joseph Janse, president of the National College of Chiropractic, in his book *Chiropractic Principles and Technique*, 2nd edition, points out that the philosophy underlying chiropractice is summed up in five principles.

(a) That a vertebra may become subluxated.

(b) That this subluxation tends to impingement of the structures, nerves, blood vessels and lymphatics passing through the intervertebral foramina.

(c) That as a result of such impingement the function of the correspondent segment of the spinal chord, and its connecting spinal and autonomic nerves, is interfered with and the conduction of the nerve impulses impaired.

(d) That as a result thereof the innovation to certain parts of the organism is abnormally altered, and such parts become functionally, or organically, diseased, or predisposed to disease.

(e) That adjustment of a subluxated vertebra removes the impingement of the structures passing through the intervertebral foramina, thus restoring to the diseased parts their normal innovation and rehabilitating them functionally and organically.

The actual procedure involved in chiropractice practice includes the following:

1. The taking of a detailed and comprehensive case history to determine all factors relating to the patient's health, to assist in the decision on the indications and contra-indications for chiropractice care.

2. Such physical examination as is necessary to further assist in this decision, with special emphasis on the spine and pelvis and the nervous system, includes a visual examination of the patient, postural study, radiography, various neurological tests and the use of various instruments to detect nerve interference.

3. The manual correction of subluxations and fixations in the human body, especially those in the spinal column and

pelvis, for the removal of interference to nerve transmission and expression as a cause of disease. This corrective procedure known as a chiropractice adjustment is a well-calculated, planned, specific thrust, applied to subluxated vertebra of the spinal column, and is a procedure which requires careful study and years of practice by the student of chiropractice, to enable him or her to become proficient, for chiropractors are most cognizant of the importance of such factor contributions to the health and hygiene of the public.

4. Rest, exercise, relaxation, education, environment, and individual conduct are necessary adjuncts.

Looking back over the years, trying to discover the reason why the science of chiropractice produced so much opposition in its early years from the dedicated men and women, of almost all the professions, whose mission in life was to help their fellow man to recover from sickness to health, I would voice the opinion of many of my colleagues oft expressed, in writings and lectures, and add them to my own, and they can all be summed up in one word—"*Simplicity*". The professional man has become accustomed over many years to the vast amount of time expended on research in any direction before the discovery of a cause and reason. The idea is almost inconceivable that anything so complicated as ill-health, which includes lack of function, lack of locomotion, lack of sensation, reduction of circulation could, in so many cases, be caused by a movement of a vertebra.

A thoroughly trained man can restore such vertebrae to their normal positions by carefully calculated, planned, specific thrusts deftly administered to the offending vertebra, pressure is released, removing interference with life force distribution to restore health. Such an idea seemed too simple and therefore quite impossible to the uninitiated.

Nevertheless, the fact remains that the extreme simplicity of one single specific cause, for one specific dis-ease with one specific correction, embracing one internal source of cure, self sufficiently contained internally within the body of the sick person, is what makes the chiropractice principle and practice so successful. No wonder the average person finds it mystifying, baffling, and difficult to understand, and probably in another way more difficult still for the professional physician.

The doctor of chiropractice who administers these adjustic thrusts to subluxated vertebrae knows that inside each of us is an innate intelligence that generates and creates all the energy needed to supply man's requirements from cradle to grave.

He knows that this generated power maintains us in health when we are well.

He knows that (if uninterrupted) it will suffice to restore us to health when we are sick.

He knows that the generated power within the brain flows from above down naturally, from brain to body, producing health.

He knows that when there is interruption, partial blockage of nerve energy compressing spinal cord or its ramifications anywhere outside of the skull, he can locate this with his scientific instruments, such as the neurocalograph and neurocalometer.

He knows he can ascertain any malposition of a vertebra with his x-ray spinograph and can and does adjust such malpositions *by hand* only, and by such adjustment release the pressure upon the nerves at the opening in the spinal column through which the nerves pass, the result of such release being restoration of normal energy, bringing about increased functions at nerve ends.

He knows all this because he is equipped to measure, calibrate, and evaluate quantity flow *before* and *after* corrective spinal adjustment.

It is a known fact that any compression of the spinal cord within the Foramen Magnum produced by a reduction of space in the neural canal, whether by faulty placement of the first cervical vertebrae in its juxta-position with the occiput, or by a subluxation of the second, which at times through strain or tear of the check ligaments around its odontoid process, allows this process to project backwards into the neural canal thus interfering with the downward and outward flow of mental impulses and produces a general slowing down of bodily activity, impairing health and at times creating functional or pathological dis-ease.

Corrective adjustments to these spinal vertebrae can and does remove these obstructions to nerve distribution and the resultant normal nerve function restores health and activity to the sick. *It is as simple as that.*

CHAPTER ELEVEN

A Statement of facts for the professions Legal, Medical and the modern student

Thomas A. Edison once stated: "The Doctor of the future will give no medicine, but will interest his patients in the care of the human frame in diet and in the cause and prevention of disease." Some doctors of medicine have for long realized that not all disease and disabilities can be corrected by medicine alone and that the science of chiropractic applied for the correction of displaced osseous tissue, particularly the spinal column, by a thoroughly trained doctor of chiropractice is absolutely essential to the recovery of some of their patients. Many, as individuals and friends of their patients, do not hesitate to send cases of herniated discs and the like to chiropractors and whilst I expect it will be some time before the medical science as an association will openly do this, I am certain that many of you will live to see this happen.

In the meantime we must expect to receive a continuation of veiled hostility from organized medicine on the one hand, whilst on the other an all-out effort is being made to absorb chiropractic principles and practice by discovering facts about nerve root involvement from spinal origin.

In November 1946, John Chapman wrote an article entitled "The Covetous Chameleon" in which he stated that while medical politicians theorate chiropractice, medical scientists work at stealing its therapy. Modern medicine has learnt a good deal from the work of Luther Burbank and other renowned botanists. Mr. Burbank and his cohorts set apart and fostered promising novelties which appeared in nature's fountain of change, and crossed one promising plant with another, sifting the result of the crossing. From these devices came such new creations in plant life as the stoneless plum and the white blackberry.

On the other hand, progressive American medical scientists, having observed the mounting successes of a non-allopathic health science whose growing popularity and effective therapy is making alarmingly deep inroads into medical practice, have adopted the basic principles of the competing science and are now watching them grow rapidly in their own field under, of course, another name—a medical name. The name of this so-called new branch of allopathy is *Physical medicine*. Except for a new handle, it is easily recognizable in part to anyone who has been indoctrinated in the natural healing arts.

Call it what they will, physical medicine is chiropractice plus, the plus including elements of physiotherapy, heat, air, light and water, initiated and long used as supplementary measures by the chiropractor, the osteopath and the naturopath.

This new departure in medical thinking, in contrast to the chiropractic mind which has been thinking in like way for the past half-century, should cause a blush to show through the thick skin of Dr. Maurice Fishbene, recently deposed official voice of the American Medical Association. He it was who fathered, and repeatedly exercised, the story that chiropractors were attempting to enter medicine through the back door. How embarrassing it must be for him now to realize that while he was pointing the finger at the chiropractor and yelling "wolf" his own fraternity were boldly breaking into the chiropractors' house and freely helping itself to the latter's valued possessions.

It is a magnitudinous paradox that the medical profession, which generally and openly denies the possibility of minor displacements of the spine as adversely affecting the health of the human body, is now propounding the self-same proposition in its description of physical medicine. The truth of that statement is substantiated by no less a personage than Dr. Howard M. Rusk, former chief of the Convalescent Division of the U.S. Army's Office of the Air Surgeon and now consultant on civilian rehabilitation for the Baroque Committee on physical medicine.

In a broadcast on adventures in science, Dr. Rusk said that the old medicine in new bottles is called physical medicine. The treatment of disease by physical methods, as distinguished from surgery, the administration of drugs and other basic practices, involves the use of heat, cold, water, massage, manipulation, electricity in various forms, exercise, occupational therapy and mechanical devices and physical retraining.

Dr. Rusk also stated that our basic belief is that they are all valuable adjuncts in both diagnosis and treatment of disease, so valuable that they warrant much research to improve and expand them, and that they should be taught to every doctor for the care of his patients. Further proof that the medical profession has been talking through its hat in denying the existence of spinal sub-luxation is advanced in an editorial on manipulative treatment in the September 1946 issue of the official publication of the American Congress of Physical Medicine.

The article, by Travell and Travell, on therapy of low back pain by manipulation, offers not only an impressive elucidation of this difficult subject but is clearly of special interest as a proof of the belief that the sacro-iliac joint can be displaced and cause a reaction of the sacral plexus whilst the subluxation lasts.

Many orthopaedic surgeons contend that the displacement of the sacro-iliac joint cannot take place as the result of stresses applied to it, but those who have had continual experience of treating low back pains must agree with the authors that many persons showing this syndrome are often immediately relieved of their main symptoms, not only as regards pain, but also by the restoration of movements previously restricted. This sudden relief of pain and disability following a successful manipulation of the lumbo sacral region surely implies that a reduction of some slight displacement has resulted.

Morton Smart emphasizes that a slipped sacro-iliac joint which has existed for a long time is almost certain to be accompanied by adhesions in the peri-articular tissues, particularly the areolar tissues, and in many cases where a manipulation has successfully restored the joint to its normal position, symptoms may continue to be present because at the same time adhesions have not been successfully freed.

He points out that manipulation of a back which has been diagnosed as a subluxated sacro-iliac joint may successfully rid the patient of all symptoms, not only because the sacro-iliac joint has been replaced, but also because a slight displacement of one of the lateral joints between the fifth lumbar and the first sacral which was clinically undiscovered has been replaced at the same time. This type of displacement, according to Morton Smart, is much more common than is usually believed, and it is difficult to differentiate between it and a displaced sacro-iliac.

Subjects with a low back pain for any length of time develop a postural lumber kyphosis, and great relief of pain follows gradual manipulation to restore the normal lumbar lordosis. The subject of manipulation, hitherto so much neglected by the medical profession, is being gradually clarified by some of these recent contributions and deserves more extensive applications, as suggested by the author. This, mind you, after more than half a century of condemnation of natural healing by the medical profession! This, too, while medical propagandists continue to work up new attacks aimed at destroying public confidence in the chiropractor, the osteopath and the naturopath.

Why this *volte-face*, this subterfuge? In the beginning, chiropractic was founded by a layman, and medical antipathy was to be expected. The manipulative arts were nothing more than fads, in the view of the medical man, who frankly was not sufficiently schooled in anatomy and physiology at that time to comprehend the importance of spinal integrity to the overall well-being of the human body.

With the raising of medical educational standards and the accruing of gigantic research funds came realization on the part of the many of the medical fraternity that chiropractic scientists were not talking through an empty hat. This was further substantiated by chiropractic success among medical casts-offs— people for whom there was declared to be no hope medically, as early as 1918.

An article by N. E. King, M.D. in *Therapeutic Review* stated, "The sooner the medical profession recognizes the work of a chiropractor the better. He is doing a work that medicine cannot do. He belongs exclusively to the class of specialists and should be so recognized."

The fame of chiropractice spread to England, and in 1924 Drs. Osgood and Morrison, in an article appearing in the *British Medical and Surgical Journal*, referred to brilliant and rapid chiropractic cures. There has been much more scientific substantiation of chiropractic in medical papers, and it is especially significant that while numerous M.D.s have switched to chiropractic in the course of the last twenty-five years, there is no known case of a chiropractor forsaking his profession for a medical degree. Despite all the obstacles put in his way, the doctor of chiropractice of today has a practice comparable to that of the M.D., a fact which is verified by both medical and chiropractic surveys on a national scale.

As a result of this economic picture, the medic who prescribed to recognizing chiropractic as a sister science was taken aside by a less altruistic, less democratic brother, who in a hypothetical discussion pointed out: "We cannot recognize chiropractic without losing face and appearing short-sighted in the eyes of the general public. You see value in the science, and wish to make use of it in your practice, either as a specific or a supplement. Remember the platitude, If the mountain won't come to Mahommed, then Mahommed must go to the mountain. There is no bar to our establishing a research programme, setting up our own schools for specialization in adjustic techniques, and offering the public physical as well as medical service in good time.

Unethical certainly, but here is more evidence of the employment of this strategy. Physiotherapy, long challenged by old line medics, was established as a special department in military hospitals during the war. The annual convention of the American Medical Association in 1942 was described by a *Times* correspondent as looking more like the chiropractic convention than a medical convention, so predominant were spinal exhibits.

The Baroque Committee on Physical Medicine has already established fellowships in various medical schools and provided funds for extensive research on manipulative therapy.

One would think that this evolution in the medical profession would have a negative effect on the chiropractor, causing him to fear the future of his science. On the contrary, the doctor of chiropractice knows that manipulation and other nature cure practices will be utilized by the medical profession as supplementary measures to surgery and drugs, and that this procedure will not bear fruit. He knows, too, that chiropractic is fifty years in advance of physical medicine as conceived by the allopath, and the rate of growing public patronage will be scientifically approved and accredited as a co-public health authority, long before the medical profession can hope to achieve the successful practice of physical medicine which will meet with public approval. The intelligent layman will reason, why wait fifty years for a health-producing article in a green wrapper when it is available now in a red one?—red that is to the old-line medical practitioner.

Among the articles submitted to the Royal Commission on Health Services in 1962 to the Canadian Government, I was particularly interested in the following:

1. How blind can Doctors be? by the London *News Chronicle*.
2. Report from the German Medical Magazine *Zeitschrift*, 1958.
3. The findings of a Harvard researcher, David David, M.D. American.

Firstly, the newspaper article—"It is fantastic that no serious attempt should have been made by the medical profession to assess the results of osteopathic and chiropractic manipulation in cases of acute and chronic backache."

The excerpts from the former London *News Chronicle* medical correspondent follow:

1. "A patient with acute backache has a poor chance of getting better quickly with the treatment generally available under the Nationalized Health Service. This is my experience as a G.P. and many people who have had slipped discs, or have strained their backs, will bear me out. Thousands of patients with backache, under whatever label, slipped disc, lumbo sacral strain, lumbago, after trailing from G.P. to Hospital and back to G.P. go eventually to an osteopath or chiro-practor outside the National Health, are manipulated and get better. The situation is ludicrous. Only a handful of doctors use these methods, and if they do they are regarded as cranks or worse by their orthodox colleagues."

Listen to *Sir Reginald Watson Jones*, the distinguished *Ortho-paedic Surgeon*, speaking about spinal manipulation at the Royal Society of Medicine:

"It is a harmful procedure no matter what the source of the low back pain may be."

To be fair to Sir Reginald he went on to stress, "*The undoubted dangers of spinal manipulation* in *unskilled hands,*" but that is not an argument against all spinal manipulation, it is only a reason for seeing that it is never performed without first making quite sure that there is no underlying disease which manipulation can make worse.

Obviously, a doctor using x-rays can be sure of this, and more than 80% of the members of the British Chiropractic Association possess their own x-ray equipment, the remainder having x-ray facilities available.

Yet what happens at present? A labourer slips and strains his back. He can neither walk nor stand without pain. His general practitioner sees him and puts him to bed for a week with hot water bottles and aspirin. At the end of that time, as he is not much better, he is given a note to attend an orthopaedic clinic. After some time he gets an appointment. There the surgeon has him x-rayed, and diagnoses a slipped disc. He calls it a *prolapsed intervertebral disc*, and puts the poor fellow into a most uncomfortable contraption called a plaster jacket. This almost immobilizes his spine, and reduces his pain, but he still cannot work.

So far, he has cost us all quite a lot of money in treatment and sick benefit. Worse is still to come. After a month the plaster jacket is removed and he is given an expensive corset, reinforced with steel, specially made for him. He still cannot walk normally. He is instructed to attend the physiotherapy department three times a week and a 32 h.p. ambulance with a crew of two carries him to and from the hospital.

After six weeks of this his acute pain has gone, but any attempt at labouring work brings back all his old symptoms. What does he do?

He returns to his family doctor, who may well admit that he can do no more. He may also scribble the name of a chiropractor on a scrap of paper and push it across his desk mumbling something like, "Don't say I sent you." Whether his National Health Service doctor sends him or not, our patient with backache frequently ends up with a chiropractor or an osteopath who clears up his symptoms.

In the clinic of one well-known chiropractor, I met three doctors' wives having treatment, and one doctor. One of the wives was brought by her own husband.

Now let us compare this with the article that appeared in 1958 from a German source. It is a translation from the German Medical Magazine *Zeitschrift* which reported on the findings of spinal abnormalities in 86 of 100 ulcer patients.

To quote, "It became more and more apparent that clinical medicine, especially internal medicine, pays too little attention to vertebral variations, and we believe it behoves every responsible physician to draw therapeutic consequences from these new findings. The application of chiropractice of course, will be indicated in almost every case because we will always find a vertebral involvement.

"It would be wrong, on the other hand, to give up completely the old, proven methods for a not entirely proven theory. We therefore originally adjusted a group of patients, mostly women, suffering from headaches, shoulder arm syndrome, and lumbago. We were amazed to find that abdominal pains of various types, of which these patients had complained for many years, had disappeared without trace.

"We then took patients who suffered from specific internal diseases, and adjusted them in the involved dorsal area. So far we have found *not one case* which failed to respond to some extent. The results often are so fantastic, that the patients believe it a miracle, and one can understand this after having been under medical care for years without results. We believe, out of personal experience, that good chiropractic must have an influence over the entire vegetative system above and beyond the local influence."

We come now to the question of chiropractic care of stomach ulcers, and various other visceral cases with spinal involvement. We must, after our experiments and research, join entirely to the idea of Gutzeit, namely, that changes in the dorsal spine, especially in diseases of the viscera, play a very important pathogenic part in diseases of the viscera. We have drawn out of these findings some therapeutic consequences.

We are often inclined to speak of real visceral disease only when we detect definite morphological findings.

Almost all nerve interference produced by the spinal column leads to functional disturbances in the viscera which we cannot detect immediately with our present diagnostic procedures. Only the heart presents the opportunity for a thorough functional diagnosis by the electrocardiograph, but it is also possible to correct heart disturbances by adjustment of the cervical vertebrae. Misalignment in the dorsal spine could be the cause of visceral disease, but the misalignment could also exercise only a localized influence, and certainly would not constitute the only pathogenic momentum.

A typical dorsal spine subluxation can cause the building up of calculii in kidney and gall bladder. Abnormal tonicity and mobility and hindered drainage, mostly easily seen in x-ray, lead to inflammation, and this, together with changes in the composition of the products to be excreted, leads to the formation of calculii.

The stomach ulcer is another example of the localized influence of abnormalities in the dorsal spine. To accept only a vertebral factor in the etiology of the stomach ulcer is not a disputable question as far as we know now.

A known malfunctioning of the vegetative system brings out a definite change in the vascular system prior to the development of the ulcer. Add to that exogenous causes, such as physic factors, which beside bringing about stomach malfunction also add capillary damage. Since vegetative and vascular abnormalities in stomach ailments are of a general nature, and not limited to the stomach, it has been a question for many years why abnormalities lead to ulceration only in the stomach and duodenal.

Only in these organs can one attach a pathogenic factor to the acid juices when conditioned tissue cells are heavily damaged by nutrition. But that nerve interference brought about in the dorsal region has an influence on production of a stomach ulcer through the vascular system is indicated by the research of F. Ditmar, who says that many marked vascular changes are produced in the outer coat of the stomach. The research of Crawl and Ryan indicate the same findings. According to Bartch, skeletal changes may cause vegetative, vascular irritation, and thereby become blood vascular reflex mechanisms.

In considering any of several visceral ailments one has the impression that the supplying of blood vessels, the tonicity and vitality of the organs, are affected by changes in the dorsal spine. *Rickers* considers changes in the nerve channels as a primary cause of disease. Is the stomach ulcer a typical example of *Rickers' neuropathological trend*?

Development of the actual ulcer occurs at the end of a series of functional disturbances which include the hormonal factor. These disturbances are in reciprocal influence with intermingling nervous and hormonal factors, but all extra vertebral and extra gastric etiological factors cannot account for stomach ulcers. When one succeeds in interrupting these disturbances emanating from the dorsal region all other etiological factors in relation to stomach ulcers are without effect.

We now come to the Harvard researchers' findings which parallel so much chiropractice, for medical practitioners and researchers are producing a growing tide of evidence and opinion which, whether they know it or not, supports the plain and simple truths of chiropractice.

In 1958, the International Review of Chiropractic quoted the research findings of *David Davis, M.D.*, an instructor in medicine at Harvard University, and a former research fellow at *Beth, Israel Hospital*, who described his discoveries (in a recently published text *"Radicular syndromes with emphasis on chest pain simulating coronorary disease"*). Dr. Davis's findings on nerve involvement greatly parallel those of *Dr. D. D. Palmer* who launched the science of chiropractice on similar premises some sixty years ago and I would therefore like to present them to you as written.

Official medicine for many years has scoffed at the idea of nerve pressure or impingement at the intervertebral foramina. The *American Medical Association*, as such, still ridicules chiropractic because of competitive economic reasons, but honest *university researches* continue to confirm the importance of the nervous system in health and sickness. Unlike the two German M.D.s who reported fantastic chiropractic results, Dr. Davis apparently made no attempt to adjust patients showing the symptoms he describes.

Following are excerpts from his text. Recognition of a disorder demands its consideration in differential diagnosis, and this is especially important in dealing with the causes of chest pain. While in over 90% of cases chest pain is due to coronary disease, spinal root compression or physiogenic disturbance must be considered if errors are to be avoided. Once one becomes alerted to the spinal root, chest pain syndromes, root compression will be found to be one of the common causes of chest pain.

Illustrating its incidence, a cardiologist is well aware of it when it is on his report of 197 cases in a survey of 600 consecutive patients complaining of chest pain. The fact it so often simulates various manifestations of coronary disease makes it a particularly important differential diagnosis.

In the vast majority of cases, root compression results from faulty body mechanics, postural or occupational strain and trauma, which in time cause the soft tissue and bony changes of osteo-arthritis of the spine. Degenerative disc disease, with or without protrusions, spurs about the posterior vertebral margins and the inter-articulate joints; deformities of the root pouch or fibrosis of a root sleeve, are conditions that most commonly produce root irritation of the chest pain. Primary neoplasm of the spinal cord and meninges and metastatic lesions from such primary sites as the prostate, lungs, or gastro-intestinal tract, may also be responsible for root compression, and these sources must be considered in diagnosis.

A rough idea of the possible role of some of these factors can be obtained from plain roetgenology and sometimes more exact information from myelography. The age, occupation, presence or absence of trauma, type of onset, duration and severity of symptoms and signs, and their response to therapy, give some information as to the probable character of the lesion.

Studies show the compression of the ventral motor roots produce pain in the distribution of the muscles supplied by these roots, and this type of pain differs in character from that due to dorsal sensory root compression.

Motor root pain is usually dull, gnawing, aching, continuous and more localized. *Sensory* root pain is *intermittent, sharp, stabbing* and frequently radiates down the upper extremities. Another form of pain more superficial in character and most often described as a tingling, or "pins and needles sensation", and frequently associated with numbness of the hands and fingers, is also of sensory root origin. Motor and sensory root pain may co-exist.

Compression of lower cervical motor roots produces pain in the region of the serratos and pectoral muscles that are innovated by these roots. The skin of the chest wall and the intercostal muscles are supplied by the upper thoracic sensory roots. Therefore chest pain may arise from either the *lower cervical, or the upper dorsal thoracic regions of the spine.*

The higher incidence of changes in the lower cervical spine in contrast to the upper thoracic, suggests that the lower cervical roots are more often the cause of symptoms; the frequent occurrence of chest pain with motor root characteristics also suggest a lower cervical origin. Chest pain due to root irritation may be mild or severe, sharp or dull, intermittent or prolonged, localized or widespread, and occur with or without radiation. When severe, it may simulate myocardial infarction, coronary failure, angina pectoris or pleurisy. More often it is a prolonged dull constricting distress that arises from the ventral motor roots irritation that suggests coronary disease.

Pain of spinal origin may occur over any part of the chest, in the back, or either side of the spine, in the axilla, in front of the breasts, and sub-sternally. Occasionally it radiates from sternum to jaws or neck region, where it may be felt as a choking sensation. Severe attacks may be accompanied by pallor and excessive perspiration; in some patients the chest pain is precipitated by walking, *simulating angina pectoris.* Many patients also complain of a peculiar respiratory distress, characterized by the inability to breathe in or out. It may be associated with other cervical root symptoms, such as shoulder girdle pain, occipital headache or vertigo.

In addition to the many features that suggest coronary disease, certain cardiacal characteristics of radicular pain are usually present. Attacks frequently occur in relation to certain movements or postures, such as bending or turning or prolonged sitting in a crouching position; after coughing, sneezing, deep breathing or straining at stool, and after hours of recumbency often waking the patient from sleep.

These relationships are not always volunteered. The patient has to be questioned to bring out this information, and sometimes significant data are obtained only when subsequent attacks are observed. The root syndrome may appear suddenly as an overwhelming attack of severe chest pain without any previous history to suggest a disorder of the spine, in a pain simulating myocardial

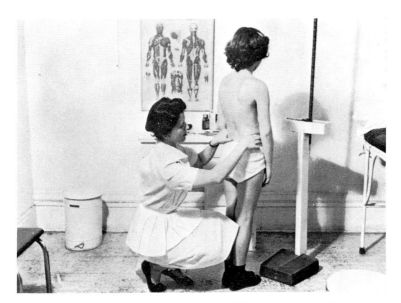

7. Checking sacral base for postural defects. (Women make excellent chiropractors, especially in the pediatric field.)

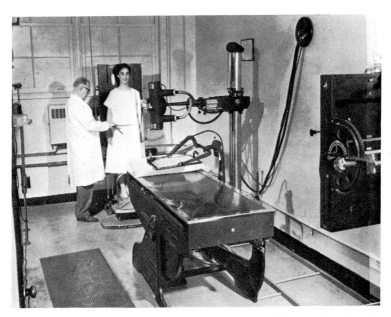

8. Preparation of a patient for spinography (x-rays of the spinal column), Canadian Memorial College, Toronto.

B.   The following photographs are taken from the pages of chiropractic and medical publications which were printed 41 years apart. A comparison of the photographs will demonstrate the tremendous influence that chiropractic successes have had in changing medical opinion.

Photos below from the book: "An Exposition of Old Moves" Palmer School of Chiropractic, 1911.

Photos below from the book: "Joint Manipulation Vol. II, The Spinal Column", by Mennell, 1952.

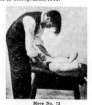

Move No. 73

Fig. 73, Page 64

EXAMINATION
OF THE
CERVICAL
AREA

Fig. 75. To show the position for examination of the cervical muscle for sensitive

Fig. 72, Page 83

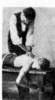

Move No. 34

Fig. 34, Page 39

SINGLE
PISIFORM
THRUST
REINFORCED

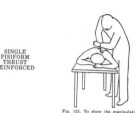

Fig. 125. To show the manipulation described in the text as the single pisiform thrust.

Fig. 125, Page 221

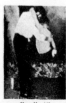

Move No. 165

Fig. 165, Page 125

LATERAL FLEXION
OF LUMBAR AND
THORACIC SPINE

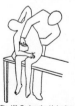

Fig. 123. To show the side-bending movement of the lumbar.

Fig. 123, Page 219

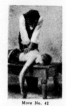

Move No. 42

Fig. 42, Page 43

DOUBLE
PISIFORM
THRUST

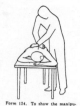

Form 124. To show the manipu-

Fig. 124, Page 220

9. Medicine approves chiropractic procedures—41 years later.

infarction. When such severe attacks are isolated, or infrequent, the cardinal characteristics of the syndrome may not be apparent.

In *root pain simulating attacks of acute coronary failure*, when such an irritation is chronic, the patient may have innumerable bouts of chest pain, lasting seconds, minutes or hours. With this number of attacks the cardinal feature of radiculitis, namely pain in relation to recumbency, positions and movements, is more likely to be apparent and this information should suggest root disease. Early in its course, however, when attacks are isolated and few in number, these relationships may not be apparent and the attacks will closely simulate acute coronary failure.

Root pains associated with respiratory distress are characterized by the inability to inspire or expire in common manifestation of lower cervical or upper thoracic root compression. Approximately one-third of patients with chest pain of root origin complain of this type of distress at some time in the course of the illness. It occurs not only with attacks of severe pain but sometimes without pain: rarely is it present in the system long before the onset of chest pain, and attacks may be sufficiently severe and persistent to suggest, erroneously, cardiac asthma.

Now root pain simulating angina pectoris, fortunately few in number, may so *closely simulate* typical angina pectoris that differential diagnosis is extremely difficult. Early in its course the chest pain may occur only in walking, or other exertion, and be relieved quickly, by rest. The type of pain may be identical in location, character and radiation with that of angina pectoris, and its occasional response to nitro-glycerine may be further misleading. Although it is seldom precipitated by excitement or cold, association with those factors is occasionally made by patients.

When the pain is induced by walking or other exertion, it must be re-emphasized that the relation is not to cardiac work performed, but to certain spinal movements that increase root irritation. Each step in walking apparently causes a little jar to the spine. particularly when the patient receives an exaggerated kyphotic posture. The absence of attacks in the same patient in the course of greater physical exertion points to a spinal factor rather than to that of angina pectoris.

Now examination for spinal tenderness. Significant tenderness over the spine at the root lesion is almost an invariable finding when symptoms of root compression are present. In the cervical region the spine should be examined for tenderness over the spinous processes, in back and over the transverse processes laterally. The upper cervical spinous processes can readily be palpated in most subjects if the neck is relaxed and in a slightly extended forward position. The transverse processes can be felt with the fingertips on each side from just below the mastoid process to the angle of the neck and shoulder. Tenderness in this region is often present when there is none over the spinous processes at the back.

Examination for tenderness should be made in various degrees, head rotation, flexion and side bending. Tenderness over the spinous processes can be elicited in the thoracic area with the ball of the thumb. In addition the thumb is placed in the groove on either side of the spinous processes, and pressure directed immediately so as to twist the vertebrae. This twisting manœuvre will sometimes evoke tenderness and referred pain to the shoulder girdle or anterior chest which is not obtained by direct pressure over the spinous processes.

In a study undertaken by the author, of 100 patients with chest pain of root origin, moderate or marked spinal tenderness was present in 94. The level of tenderness generally corresponded to the distribution of root pain with reproduction of referred pain by pressure over the spinal lesion. In 33 out of 100 patients, pressure directed over the vertebrae induced pain over the anterior or lateral region of the chest wall. Induction or relief of symptoms by movements, when a patient states that a specific body movement involving the spine induces chest pain, or that pain can be relieved by a given body position, should be *reproduced and observed*. When active movements do not induce pain, passive movements may do so and should be tried.

PART TWO

J. J. Janse's text, outlines
five principles & Technique
of Chiropractic Science
with quotes from authorative
medical writings

Much opposition to the science of chiropractice could be found in the writings of medical doctors of the past, and, possibly, one of the most outright rejections of our principles was typified in the statement by Dr. Maurice Fishbein, former editor of the Journal of the American Medical Association, when he wrote, in 1932, in his book *Fads and Quackery in Healing* (republished over his name in December 1946 by Readerscope Magazine): "The x-ray has been used to search for the dislocations which the chiropractors assert are present, but these dislocations cannot be found. Moreover, experiments conducted in California have shown that a force of 1,200 to 1,300 lbs, while it will fracture one of the spinal bones, will not dislocate it or cause it to press on the spinal nerves. Thus the fundamental dogma of chiropractice that disease is caused by dislocation or subluxations of the bones of the spinal column pressing on nerves is simply a complete mis-representation of the demonstable facts."

This erroneous view, and other similar opinions, have formed the basis for organized medical opposition to regulatory chiro-practice legislation over the years. Such opposition is in direct conflict with the public interests, and we shall deal with this subject in more detail later.

In oder to refute Dr. Fishbein's remarks with statements by his own professional colleagues, we shall repeat here the five basic principles upon which our profession is founded, and follow each with a series of supporting statements from medical authorities.

The five principles are as outlined in J. J. Janse's text "Chiro-practic principles and technique".

1. *That a vertebrae may become subluxated*
   Supporting statement:

   (a) From *Back Pain.* by John M. Mennell, M.D. Exhibit 12. Littlebrown and Company.
   "The concept of the joint lock envisages one of two things, either an unreduced sub-critical subluxation of the joint or the seizing up of its articular surfaces on one another."

   (b) D. Hoyt Cox, in his papers, "Manipulation in low back conditions, from the archives of Physical Therapy", January 1935, Exhibit 13, *Medicine and Chiropractic,* page 20, speaking on the possibility of sacro-iliac sub-luxation states: "Evidence that definite displacement does occur have been amply provided by the research of Goldthwaite, Osgood, Albi, Tych, Dunlop, Magnerson and Pitfield."

(c) Dr. F. A. Jostice, eminent American Orthopaedist, in an article "Neck pain, the laminagraph as an aid to the diagnosis of atlanto-occipital lesions", Journal of the American Medical Association, Volume 118 No. 8 1942, Exhibit 13, *Medicine and Chiropractic*, page 33, states:
"The occipital condyles may be displaced on the atlas so that there exists an atlanto-occipital subluxation."

(d) D. James P. Woddersee in *Surgical Treatment*, Vol. 1, page 623, states:
"Subluxations of vertebrae occur in all parts of the spine and in all degrees. When the dislocation is so slight as not to affect the spinal cord it will still produce disturbances in the spinal nerves passing off through the spinal foramina."

(e) Dr. Edgar Cyriax, noted British Orthopaedic Surgeon, in his collected papers on Therapeutics, London, 1924, Exhibit 13, *Medicine and Chiropractic*, page 38, states:
"It appears that the medical profession while frankly admitting that minor displacements of bones and cartilages in the extremities can arise and be reduced, refuse to hold these views as regards the vertebral column. Up to the present, however, none of those who hold these opinions have been able to give me one reason in support of their statements." It will be noted in a later reference through Dr. Edgar Cyriax's present activities, that much of which he has stated there, has changed so considerably that vertebral adjustments are common practice in his and associates' surgeries.

(f) In the Journal of the American Medical Association, Volume 104, pages 1578 in 1935, Stimpson and Swenson, of the staff of the Presbyterian Hospital of New York, reported: "Since 1st January 1929 there have been 66 cases of unilateral subluxation of the cervical vertebrae without associated fracture seen in the Fracture

Service of Presbyterian Hospital. Of these, five were seen in the first three years, and 39 cases in the past 18 months.

"This sudden and spectacular increase is not due to any change in the neck structure of New York's population, but to the education of the members of the staff in recognition of the condition." The report goes on to describe the nature of the subluxations, and is quoted more extensively in *Medicine and Chiropractic*, Exhibit 13, pages 32 and 33.

2. That this subluxation tends to impingement of the structures (on nerves, blood vessels, and lymphatics) passing through the intervertebral foramina.

Supporting statements:

(a) Dr. Paul C. Williams. "Reduced lumbo-sacral joint space, Journal of the American Medical Association, 12th November 1932. Exhibit 13, Medicine and Chiropractic, page 23. In this article Dr. Williams designates subluxation of the fifth lumbar vertebra as one of the causes of reduced lumbo-sacral joint space, and consequent nerve irritation.

(b) D. A. Kovaks. "Subluxation and Deformation on a cervical apophyseal joint. *Contribution to the Etiology of Headache*". *Medicine and Chiropractic*, Exhibit 13, page 34. In reviewing this article for a Radiology magazine Lawrence A. Pillar states: "In this paper the author deals with the subluxations of the small joints of the upper cervical spine which results in constriction of circulatory disturbance in the vertebral artery, and impaired function of the sympathetic vertebral plexus. The artery and nerve are rather frequently affected by the deformities of adjacent borders, bilateral or unilateral headaches result; headache radiating from the top of the skull and the nucal region is more frequently produced by pressure on the vertebral artery and nerve than in any other condition."

(c) D. O. B. Chamberlain. Cervical Arthritis. Journal of the South Carolina Medical Association 1942. Exhibit 13, *Medicine and Chiropractic*, page 42.

"This is the important point, that the sensory nerve roots before they get out of the foramina and form nerves, may be pressed upon by various bones and soft tissue changes."

(d) Drs. E. L. Turner and A. Oppenheimer in "Annals of Internal Medicine", October 1937, Exhibit 13, *Medicine and Chiropractic*, page 42.

"If one studies the relationship of the intervertebral foramina through which the nerves pass as they leave the spinal canal in the cervical region, it is quite obvious that narrowing of the inter-spaces between the vertebrae can, and does, change the diameter of the foramina."

3. That as a result of such impingement the functions of the corresponding segment of the spinal cord and its connecting spinal and autonomic nerves is interfered with and *the conduction of the nerve impulses impaired*.

Supporting statements:

(a) *Back Pain* by John M. Mennell, M.D., pages 15 and 16. Exhibit 12. "Conversely, another most dramatic case comes to mind of a patient who for many years had suffered from severe angina pectoris. Then, one day, an astute cardiologist satisfied both the patient and her family doctor that her heart was perfectly sound. Examination revealed gross impairment of movement in the joints of the thoracic spine between the 3rd and 6th thoracic vertebra. Restoration of normal movement in these joints relieved the patient's pain which for all this time had been erroneously diagnosed as coming from within the heart instead of as referred pain in the pre-cordial structures of the chest wall in front of the heart."

(b) Dr. James B. Wardessee. Article entitled "Dislocations of cervical vertebrae" in the American Journal of Surgery, March 1909, Exhibit 13, *Medicine and Chiropractic*, page 42, said:

"Dislocations of cervical vertebrae vary in degree. The most common are the slight subluxations which produce no pressure on the cord, which give rise to more or less local discomfort, and which are important because the distortion is often great enough to cause pressure upon the spinal nerves passing out between the vertebrae. This pressure or irritation of the nerve trunks in these more common cases causes nerve disturbances which are referred remotely from the site of the lesion, namely, at the peripheral distribution of the nerves, and are manifested as peripheral pain, muscular weakness, or trophic derangements."

(c) The Journal of the American Medical Association was quoted by the News Service of the National Chiropractic Association in September 1961 as follows:

Exhibit 15. C.C.A. Journal, Volume 5, No. 5, Page 3, says: "*Pain around the heart,* even when agonizing and of a constricting nature, and radiating down the left arm, may be caused by trouble in the spine instead of the *heart disease angina pectoris,* which it resembles." *Note.* (Angina pectoris is a simple heart disease and not a disease in itself.)

Colonel Alan Isord Jose and Lieut. Colonel Francis Murphy of the O'Reilly General Hospital at Springfield, Missouri, report:

"*The spinal trouble* which they found causing the pain in 30 cases *was due to a narrowing of the intervertebral foramina,* of the upper dorsal vertebrae as produced by vertebral shifting. The Army Medical Officers believe from their experience that upper dorsal vertebral shifting should be conjectured in all cases suspected of having either angina pectoris or coronary occlusion, in whom the symptoms, physical signs and laboratory examinations are not conclusive."

4. Again, in J. J. Jansen's text, "Chiropractic Principles and Technique", (that as the result of spinal vertebral subluxations the innovation to certain parts of the organism is abnormally altered and such parts become functionally or organically diseased or pre-disposed to disease).
Supporting statements:

(a) In essentials of body mechanics by the following authors: Joel E. Goldthwaite, M.D., F.A.C.S., LL.D.; Lloyd T. Brown, M.D., F.A.C.S.; Laurel T. Swain, M.D.; John

G. Gunns, M.D., F.A.C.S.; William J. Kerr, M.D., F.A.C.P. Exhibit 16. It is stated on page 45: "It is possible to have irritation at the spinal roots in this region (dorsal lumbar spine) with accompanying referred pain in the abdomen. It is beginning to be realized that many of the painful symptoms in the region of the appendix, lower abdomen, and gall bladder may be due to this cause rather than to any pathology in the viscera themselves."

(b) The authors on page 110 state: "In many instances there is a similar distribution of pain, and a diagnosis of angina pectoris is wrongly made where there is no disturbance to the circulation of the musculature of the heart. The electrocardiograph shows no evidence of such disturbance. Here the cause of the pain is the irritation of the lower cervical and upper thoracic nerves. This is brought about by faulty body mechanics through pressure on or pinching of the nerves, either at their foramina of exit or at the costal vertebral joints. This is produced through the increased flexion of the spine, the downward displacement of the ribs, and the over-stretching of spinal muscles and ligaments. Impingement of the nerves can occur much more easily if there is an arthritis about the spinal joints."

Again, the authors state, on page 184: "There is, however, another type of nerve root irritation showing similar pathology and functional disturbances due to mechanical causes, usually the result of pressure or stretching of the nerve roots. The many joints and bony processes about the spine, and the numerous ligaments and muscular attachments make the spinal nerve roots peculiarly liable to mechanical irritation. Examples of this have been found by many observers in radiating pains about the shoulder girdle and in the arms, and in such pains as sciatica in the lower extremities. The same observers have noted the disappearance of the pain after the correction of the faulty body mechanics. Garnett and Gunther have described the frequent occurrence of symptoms which simulate the cerebral disease, particularly that of the gall bladder and appendix. They disappeared with the removal of the mechanical irritation."

Dr. George S. Weiger, in his book *Genesis and Control of Disease*, said: "When skeletal abnormalities exist, be they ever so slight or apparently trivial, we must admit that either directly, or indirectly, they affect muscles or organs through pressure on nerves or ganglia. We cannot deny anything which irritates a nerve or ganglia or interferes in any way with the free flow of nerve force to the parts supplied may readily disturb the function of that part of give rise to pain in the nerve trunk itself or in the peripheral organ. Unrelieved functional disturbances eventually lead to organic changes."

The fifth Chiropractic principle that adjustment of a subluxated vertebrae removes the impingement of the structures is supported by Dr. J. H. Radley. In *Medicine and Chiropractic*, page 39 (listed in "Who's Who in American Medicine") he stated in 1914 that spinal subluxations are a frequent occurrence, that they attend if they do not precede and cause disease in remote tissue, and that correction of these lesions is followed by restoration to normal conditions and functions of such remote tissue are all matters of repeatedly demonstrated fact.

Again, Dr. T. D. Stam in "Role of Manipulation in lower back pain" from Guy's Hospital, London, Exhibit 13, *Medicine and Chiropractic*, page 52 in July 1934 said: "*In subluxation*, manipulation affords the only rational treatment, and gives satisfactory results. In chronic strain the adhesions can be broken down by manipulation and full mobility restored. Manipulation is often followed by considerable relief of pain."

Dr. Frimort Beiderman in *Fundamentals of Chiropractic* from the standpoint of a medical doctor says: "Six months after fracture of the surgical neck of the right humerus the patient had only very limited motion and shoulder articulation. Running and exercise and many other therapies improve the situation only very slightly, but *one spinal adjustment in the cervical region immediately and permanently restored the motion in the shoulder joint*, and reduced to a minimum the radiating pains in the upper right arm. In a few days results were complete following this segmental therapy."

The foregoing evidence from medical sources, supporting the five basic principles of the chiropractice profession is covered in more complete detail in the book *Medicine and Chiropractic* by Weiant and Goldschimpt.

Many interesting examples of duplicity can be found by comparing photos from the book, *an exposition of old moves (Palmer Chiropractic College 1911)* with those published in the book *Joint Manipulation, Volume 2, The Spinal Column* by Mennell 1952, thus proving that *medicine approves chiropractice procedures forty-one years later.*

The preceding photographs were taken from the pages of chiropractic and medical publications which were printed forty-one years apart. The comparison of the photographs will demonstrate the tremendous influence that chiropractice successes have had in changing medical opinion.

CHAPTER TWELVE

A Spot of Research

Thirty years ago at Palmer College we were busy researching into the occipital atlanto axial region of the cervical spine. As we found that more spectacular recoveries from disease and disability responded from spinal adjustments in this region, and very much quicker than any other part of the spinal column, B. J. Palmer, the developer of the science, practically ceased making any other adjustments to the spinal column except occipital atlas and axis.

In this region there were no osseous locking devices to check the atlas moving under severe strain sidewise off the condyles of the occiput and also with a degree of rotation. The check ligaments around the odontoid of axis were the only restrictive means of preventing a partial occlusion of the neuro canal by the odontoid.

In addition, we had a reduction of the foramen magnum by the atlas above, side-slipping either right or left with an additional rotation to the anterior or posterior. Then we had found a major cause of much disease by the reduction of the flow of mental impulses from the brain through the spinal cord to all parts of the body.

Our elation, however, was short-lived, in that from all sources we were met with the facts quoted by many of our own profession, and equally from many medical colleges and research centres, that dissection had proved that the foramen magnum was too large, the spinal cord was too small. These groups set the hypothesis that an atlas could not in any sense produce pressure upon the spinal cord, because of the fact that the spinal cord was only about the size of a cigarette, that it rattled around in a great big hole, that the bone could only move a certain degree, that the hole was a great big one, and also a spinal cord the size of a cigarette was too small to be subjected to pressure because of the size of the hole.

B. J. Palmer spoke of that, not in a personal sense, not in a pre-
judicial sense, but because he felt that we are all more or less
interested in the facts.

Now what are the scientific facts? I quote from Palmer.

"I say that if the theory advanced were sound, that the spinal
cord at the atlas, or anywhere in the neurocanal, was so small that
no ordinary subluxation, wrench or movement would or could
produce a pressure upon the spinal cord, then obviously we would
have consistently to dig up the medical hypothesis of anatomy.
That the nerves as they issue through the intervertebral foramina
are of themselves in ratio of so small a size that no ordinary subluxation, wrench or movement of any of the vertebrae could produce
any pressure upon any of them, and, if that held good, then chiropractice was and has been all through the years a fraud, and the
atlas work was on a theory that could not, and would not, hold
water. That was the only conclusion that could be reached if the
hypothesis were correct as a matter of science."

This, then, brought another phase of work that had to be gone
into most carefully. We had to find out whether the spinal cord
was the size of a cigarette, and was it impossible for a vertebra
to be subluxated and thereby produce pressure upon the spinal
cord, because it was so small that it rattled around in this great
big hole called the neuro-canal.

The first move made by B. J. Palmer to discover the actual size
of the spinal cord in the foramen magnum was a visit to a research
laboratory in the U.S.A. There he talked over methods of ascer-
taining the relative size of the cord in relation to the structure in
which it was presumed to be at its largest, and all agreed that the
region was the occipital atlanto axial one.

Now the Professor of the research laboratory said to him,
"Anything we may have here to help you, is at your command.
You may do anything you want, but what you want you won't
get, because to obtain this you need a cadaver, practically immediately after death. While time elements vary from State to
State, on average the earliest it would be possible to obtain an
unclaimed cadaver would be about eight to twelve months.'

The conversation between the two great men continued as
follows:

The Professor in charge of the research laboratory said, "In the first place a vertebral subluxation is a rare thing, and in the second place, even if it did exist as you say, you still would not find what you want to find, because there would be no pressure there."

"Professor," said B. J. Palmer, "that is the very matter, the very problem in dispute. If you are right I want to know it, but I do not want it as a matter of opinion. I want it as a matter of proof. Now let us both throw our theories and our opinions of controversial things away, and let us prove whether you are right or I am right."

The Professor said, "I am perfectly willing to do that, but what you want you still won't get."

"Why, Professor?" B. J. Palmer again asked him.

He said, "I will tell you why. Because at the very moment of death every tissue in the body begins shrinking within 24 hours. Your spinal cord has shrunk just 50 % in circumference and diameter. Within 48 hours this has stepped up to within 60% shrinkage, and the longer the body lays embalmed the more it goes on shrinking with the spinal cord producing by far the greatest shrinkage of any of the tissue structures of the body. All tissues shrink, but where the muscles may shrink 5% in two years, your spinal cord would have shrunk 80%, and you would have lost 80 % of your claimed pressure upon the spinal cord due, as you state, to a subluxation of the vertebrae, so that 80% of what you want to show is not any longer there."

B. J. Palmer then said, "I see that I am foiled; I cannot prove it here, so I will go to Germany."

In Germany he found that if you could convince the Government that there was something in a phase of research that you want to undertake, they would give you a special permit to do the new research work.

After putting this proposition to the proper authorities, they said, "We stand ready to carry out your exacting scientific stipulation." He explained that he wanted to ascertain whether an atlas subluxation does, or does not, produce pressure upon a spinal cord that has not shrunk and cannot shrink.

He said, to the great German professor (who made all the dissections for the spalteholtz anatomy), "In your profession, Professor, in your research work here in your laboratory, do you agree with our professors in the United States, that the spinal cord shrinks 50% in 24 hours?"

He said, "No, I do not. Our research here shows that the spinal cord shrinks approximately 35% in 24 hours and it take 48 hours to get to 50%. Now in Room 5 you will find 27 photographs of 27 methods of dissection that have been performed in Germany under these conditions. Some of them were on bodies embalmed for three years, some for two, some for only six months, and some immediately after death, so that by examination you will get a fair and just comparison in these photographs, which reveal the fact that the spinal cord in living man is not the size of a cigarette."

This research work proved the rule that atlas subluxation *does produce pressure upon the spinal cord*, evidence of spinal cord compression being witnessed through the courtesy of the Research Department of the German Government Medical Section.

Some real evidence must always be at hand, because words and photographs alone could not, and would not, silence those who had so emphatically denied the existence of pressure upon the spinal cord. Yet without such a condition existing, there is no basis in scientific fact that we, as doctors of chiropractice, could maintain and prove that the removal of such pressure by spinal adjustments could, and would, get sick people well.

In brief then, B. J. Palmer first obtained spinograph x-rays of the spinal column taken anterior to posterior laterally and stereo-scopically, of a person within whom a surmised compression of spinal cord existed because of the pronounced subluxation of the atlas vertebrae laterally and anteriorly, and who in addition was within the last 48 hours of the end of his life.

He requested that the immediate preservation of this section of the cervical spine be secured by the freezing method for dissection and the segments anchored as they existed during life so that the subluxation would be preserved in death. This was done, and the specimen was then put through the famous Spalteheltz process of dissolution of all the osseous, inorganic structure, leaving the organic only, leaving out the mineral elements, so that it would make possible a transparency of the occiput, atlas and axis in order that we might look through from above and see the position assumed by the occiput and atlas, and atlas upon axis, that existed as a subluxation during life, and at the time of death.

This was done in an attempt to solve a crucial question of today, one that is vitally important to us, that is, if it is fundamentally true that a man *did* die of a side-slipped atlas, that was in reality subluxated, and not merely as a matter of theory or hypothesis.

It took almost a year to dissolve that specimen and it is now hanging in a jar of formaldehyde at the Palmer College of Chiropractic. It is absolutely transparent from above downwards, or from below upwards, according from which side of the jar you look at it.

You can look right through that specimen and see the vertebrae as carried in life. It is the only specimen of its kind in the world and to our knowledge the only one that has ever been made.

To the student or doctor who is privileged to observe it, it will be noticed that it shows a definite atlas side-slipped to the left off its condyles. It is superior at its anterior and is anchored in its exact position as it was at the moment of death.

We owe a great deal to Dr. Spalteholtz, for it was only his method of dissolution that made the experiment a success. In that year, 1934, Germany was the only place in the world where this process of dissolution could be done, either by Dr. Spalteholtz himself, or under his direct supervision. Dr. Spalteholtz is also the author of *The Spalteholtz Anatomy*.

The year 1934, therefore, became an important milestone in our journey. B. J. Palmer, the developer of chiropractice, attended and addressed us at the convention of The British Chiropractic Association in London, England. We went to Germany, establishing scientific proof of actual spinal cord pressure by methods which established a protection against distortion, *supplied by Medical Science*, and finally it was the year when I decided to dispose of my Canadian practice and settled down to building another in East Anglia.

PART TWO

A little over ten years ago, specific inquiries by insurance men regarding the effectiveness of chiropractic care were undertaken following complaints by claims adjusters that lengthy convalescence and complete recoveries under medical care, especially when surgery was employed, were causing considerable concern.

The Research Department of the International Chiropractors' Association carried out an exhaustive study of about a thousand cases supplied by their members over a period of three years. It was published in booklet form entitled, *A study of 1,000 herniated and slipped discs"*; but let us quote the articles as they apply to this type of painful disability, which in paragraph 3 states:

To appreciate the chiropractic procedure one must understand that the intervertebral disc grossly consists of an outside capsule (annulus fibrosus) which, normally, is a tough white fibrous tissue holding an elastic pulpy mass (nucleus pulposus). It functions as a shock absorber, as a cartilage pad holding the vertebrae apart, and as a ligament holding them together. The structure normally allows for great flexibility of the spine, while maintaining the bodies of the vertebrae in good alignment regardless of the position of the body. Herniation involves the bulging of the annulus fibrosus so that the disc fails to perform its proper function.

Because of the normal toughness of this tissue (annulus fibrosus) the only three probable causes for true herniation or rupturing of the disc are:

1. Great TRAUMATIC Force, such as a fall from a high level. The force which would produce herniation of normal tissue would almost certainly produce a vertebrae subluxation as well. Chiropractic procedure to reduce possible subluxation is indicated.

2. PATHOLOGICAL weakness of the disc resulting from diminished nerve energy supply. Vertebral interference can cause thinning or weakening of the capsule wall to the degree that a spontaneous bulging or herniation of the central pulpy mass is produced.

3. PATHOLOGICAL weakness coupled with TRAUMA. When pathological weakness is present, complete recovery is not possible unless the tissue regains its normal toughness. Having assumed an abnormal pathological state because of failure to receive normal nerve energy supply, it follows that it cannot return to normalcy until the vertebral interference is corrected. While, in extreme cases, surgical intervention may be necessary this type of case is rare.

There is much evidence that diagnosis of "slipped disc" is a catch-all for many low back disabilities not otherwise explainable according to present medical concepts. In fact there is much to indicate that most so-called "herniated disc syndromes" are nothing more than vertebral subluxations. The statistics contained show rapid recovery in the majority of cases.

We believe that such quick recovery would not have been possible if extensive pathology or severe trauma had been present. Nevertheless, 483 of the cases reported were medically diagnosed as "herniated disc or ruptured disc" and the remaining cases manifested the same outward symptoms. Since such a diagnosis can be confirmed only by surgery, and since few symptomatically diagnosed cases are later confirmed upon surgical intervention, it would seem all the more important that a suspected case of herniated disc be referred to a chiropractor in the first instance.

The research department stated that the general public is hearing more and more about the slipped or herniated inter-vertebral disc because it is being talked and written about more often by members of the medical profession. It would almost seem that the herniated disc is now having its innings. Because of its seeming popularity, we know that this study will have far-reaching effects as it deals with *1,000 medically diagnosed* or symptomatic cases of herniated or slipped inter-vertebral disc under chiropractic care. The results of the research on this type of case under Chiropractic care are very encouraging. The study revealed that 49·6% *became well*, 39·1% were *much improved*, 7·9% were *slightly improved* and only 0·4% became worse. Consolidating the first three groups we find that 96·6% of all the cases became well or showed some improvement under chiropractic care.

The study reminds us once again that the sooner cases report to a chiropractor, the more complete their results will be, for it revealed that in the groups which *became well* (49·6% of all cases) the average length of time the condition previously existed was only 3·5 years. Whereas in those cases in which there was no change in the condition (3·0% of all cases), the average length of time was 5·5 years.

PART THREE

It is strange to look back over the years and remember the time
when the medical profession of the North American continent
openly stated that the adjustment of a subluxated vertebra by hand
was impossible, that chiropractic had no scientific basis in fact,
and sought by legal means to prevent the graduate of the first
School of Chiropractice from obtaining a licence to practise.

In many states legal action was actually taken against many of
the early pioneers of chiropractic under hastily enacted state laws
accusing them of "Practising Medicine without a Licence". Many
were fined, many others were actually put into jail. Finally public
opinion revolted against the injustice, the laws were repealed
and State Boards created consisting of a panel of medical doctors,
and doctors of chiropractice with an independent casting vote
by one not connected with either party. The State Board examination became a factor in establishing the knowledge and efficiency
of the chiropractor who was then licensed to practise his science
and enjoy the full privileges and protection of the law.

There followed the blessing of the federal government, which
included the science in the list of professions allocated under the
re-establishment and rehabilitation programme for returned
G.I.s. Insurance companies and workmen's compensations
followed in many cases when it came to be appreciated that the
time of convalescence of many cases of spinal disorder were
considerably shortened, and quicker return to employment
became possible.

Over the years we have seen a considerable change in the
attitude of the medical profession of many countries to the correction of disabilities by spinal manipulations, probably not so much
as a group of Medical Associates, but by the advanced thinking
individual M.D. This is quite understandable, for many of the
finest discoveries of medical science were not given the acknowledgement they warranted for many years—often after the discoverer had departed this world. The association, like the art
critics over the years, loudly applaud the efforts of the individual
and scientist, when such encouragement is no longer required.

However, it is now acknowledged that the much derided spinal
adjustment of the subluxated vertebrae performed many years

ago by the pioneers of our science has proved not only a possibility but an acknowledged fact, as evidenced by articles appearing from time to time in the medical journals. One hears quite often of a patient being manipulated under anaesthetics, a method tested and discarded years ago as being quite ineffective in the correction of subluxated vertebrae. This was because a rapid contraction of muscle is essential following a recoil of vertebrae in motion set up by the adjustic thrust given at the time of vertebral positional correction, and this is not possible during anaesthesia.

Personally, I have yet to be able successfully to adjust the spine of anyone under the influence of drugs, or alcohol. Again it should be here stated that seldom is it necessary to deaden sensory nerves, as a properly trained doctor of chiropractic is taught how to adjust spinal vertebrae without pain.

In some of the following paragraphs reference will frequently be made to the word 'Syndrome', meaning a number of symptoms occurring together constituting a distinct clinical picture, such as a disc syndrome, a painful back syndrome, a fifth lumbar vertebrae syndrome, etc. References such as these are frequently seen.

In an article, "Back pain and Hyperaesthesia" in *The Lancet* of 28th May 1960, the writer explained in great detail the results of his investigation of over two hundred cases of back pains, such as lumbago, sacro-iliac syndrome, sciatica and coccygeal syndrome. Mention was made that back pain is poorly understood but that the unnecessary pain (resulting in loss of man-hours) can be localized accurately and treated by manipulation without anaesthesia.

The author continued with the statement that the syndrome of pressure on a nerve root by a protruded intervertebral disc is rare in industrial practice, but that a different syndrome arose at any spinal level from occiput (base of head) to the coccyx (rudimentary tail bone) comprising a clearly defined area of hyperaesthesia (excessive sensitiveness) adjacent to the spine. A localized tender spot was associated with it, plus a dull ache in this area accompanied by limitation of movement of the trunk by reason of the pain.

This well-defined syndrome can be elicited in a large majority of cases which are usually described as torticollis, fibrositis, pleurodynia, myalgia, lumbago, and in some cases of sciatica or coccydynia (pain in the coccyx) or tail bone. The whole report was handled with extreme thoroughness and sincerity, and merits much admiration.

It is a pity, though, that the writer of this article had not delved down into the textbooks of B. J. Palmer. It would have saved many valuable hours of study and research that could have been used to advantage in embracing adjustment technique. The resultant "click" which appeared to me to evidence some surprise on the part of the investigator, ceased to surprise the *doctors of chiropractice* fifty years ago.

In 1962 the *Encylopaedia Britannica* gave the following definitions of chiropractice and osteopathy:

"Oesteopathy—the doctrine that all diseases are due to abnormalities in or near joints and that the treatment for every disease is the correction of these abnormalities without the use of drugs."

By comparison—definition of chiropractice. "A system of treatment of human disease and injuries based on the premise that the nerve system controls all other systems and all physiological functions in the body. The chiropractor treats by adjustments and manipulation of the structures of the body, especially the spinal column, to restore normal nerve function. D. D. Palmer began the practice of chiropractic in 1895."

Osteopathy, like chiropractic, has had much criticism from orthodox medicine over the years, possibly more so in view of the fact that in some instances much that belongs to *material medica* crept into the ranks of the osteopaths, principally by those not too well versed in the applications of their profession as laid down by its founder D. Andrew Still and, in my opinion, this is the major reason for the decline in its popularity.

I was, therefore, astounded to see the turn of the tables, as outlined in a book published in 1960 under the title *Disc Lesions*, in which the terminology used in many descriptions of body movements is so very similar to osteopathic terms. The illustrations of nearly all manipulatory moves to spine and pelvis (with the exception of the mechanical traction) are obviously copied from osteopathic textbooks, or have been obtained from an osteopath. 1960 appears to have been the year when chiropractic and osteopathy were acknowledged by the M.D. as essential to health in many specialized cases, and we hope that this interest increases to the extent that those who feel adaptive to specific spinal adjusting will enrol at an accredited chiropractic college, and learn its *scientific application* instead of using hit-or-miss methods of correcting misaligned or displaced vertebrae without previous training which, I regret to say, exists to a marked degree in this country.

We find this in the ranks of masseurs, the physiotherapists, some naturopaths, and self-styled osteopaths, who have not had previous training in specific spinal adjusting and, alas, some members of the medical association are using their own version of this in their general practice, with sometimes unhappy results. It is, therefore, very important to ascertain that those whom you consult about chiropractic care are fully trained and their ability acknowledged by the profession.

PART FOUR

Proof of Chemical Changes following Spinal Adjustments

Some years ago I had the privilege of meeting a man who had built up a fine reputation as an author and as an osteopath, and one who loved to delve into research of the many fields that were directly or indirectly connected with the health of man. It was, therefore, quite natural that he would be interested in the chemical changes that occur following specific spinal adjustments, and I feel sure that much of his knowledge of specific spinal adjusting was the direct result of many pleasant hours investigating chiropractice in our respective homes.

Over the years I noted a gradual swing away from many of the osteopathic methods and much substitution of specific adjusting that had proved so successful in my own practice. It was, therefore, not surprising to see much reference to the science of chiropractice in his early book *Healing Hands* and, as some remarks of mine were quoted, by name, I feel sure that he will permit me to make a few references and quotations from his recent booklet *The role of the Chemical Mediator in Spinal Manipulation*, just to even up the score. I refer, of course, to the well-known Parnell Bradbury of Hove, the best chiropractor who ever graduated from an *osteopathic school*.

In part one he states: "The chiropractor recognizes the value of preliminary soft tissue treatment in certain cases, the osteopath has recognized the significance of the specific positional subluxation. He is no longer contemptuous of the chiropractor who adjusts upper cervical vertebrae in certain cases of low backache. Clinical evidence that this method often cures the condition is irrefutable. Thousands upon thousands of patients can testify to its truth. *As Jocelyn Proby* so aptly put it at a recent meeting of osteopaths—'The group lesion of diminished mobility is more common, but the positional one is more significant'."

A research with Dr. Dudley Dee and Parnell Bradbury was first undertaken eight years ago in an attempt to prove or disprove nerve pressure theory (that is, the theory that vertebral misplacement causes nerve pressure or directly interferes with normal trnsmission of nerve impulses. Also, the claims from responsible chiropractic quarters, to the effect that cord pressure could exist in the foramen magnum region, that is the upper cervical or neck vertebrae, by a side-slipped atlas vertebrae possibly caused by some form of accident which created a whiplash recoil between vertebrae and base of occiput (posterior inferior portion of the skull). The whole set-up seemed untenable, and yet spectacular results were achieved by those working on these premises.

How? It was reasonable to suppose that certain spinal adjustments triggered off a chemical mediator. "This possibility was first suggested by the pioneer work of Elliott (1905) on medulli-adrenal secretion" wrote Albert Kuntz in his book *The Autonomic Nervous System.*

Parnell goes on to relate, "When I was in Switzerland in 1947, M. Regle, of Berne, provided me with details of a patient suffering from a serious blood condition following an accident, whom he had treated by an adjustment of the atlas (first cervical vertebra) alone. No one could have given me a more valuable clue to start my investigations.

"This patient, two years previously, sustained a double fracture of the lower leg (that is the tibia and fibula) while ski-ing in Switzerland. For eight months the usual medico-surgical treatment had been given, which included the use of traction and weights.

X-rays revealed that the bones were not knitting together and, to complicate matters, the limb was becoming gangrenous. Amputation was advised as the only means of saving the patient's life. This desperate measure drove the man to seek the services of a doctor of chiropractice (*M. Regli, D.C.*) who made the usual spinographs (x-rays of spinal vertebrae) and over a period of eight weeks made three adjustments to the first cervical vertebra. The bones began to knit up very quickly after this, and to cut a long story short, within a matter of months the leg was not only saved from amputation but the man was able to ski again.

"Such results from adjustments of spinal articulations accrue, in my opinion, from chemical mediation which follow close in the wake of waves of depolarization passing along nerve fibres which have been activated by *the adjustment*, at a given spinal segment."

Parnell Bradbury continues: "After my return to England I got in touch with Dr. Dee, whom I had known for some years, and asked him if he thought it would be possible to detect changes in the chemistry of a patient's blood after an adjustment to the spine. He was definitely of the opinion that this could be done.

"Laboratory tests were made on patients selected because pronounced subluxation of the atlas or axis vertebrae were evident, and which were, in my opinion, the major specific lesion.

"These tests, which we called the *Sympathin Test*, were carried out briefly as follows:

"Selected patients were instructed to abstain from food for two hours before the test, and not partake of any severe exertion. Then a rest period of up to thirty minutes was enforced before the taking of the first sample. A pre-adjustment blood sample followed, usually from an antecubital vein, but occasionally capillary blood was collected from the lobe of the ear or from a finger.

"*A specific spinal adjustment* was then made on the major subluxation, and the patient was immediately put to rest in the supine position. After twenty minutes' rest the second of post-adjustment blood sample was taken by the same procedure as the first.

"The 'true blood sugar' level of both samples was then compared. We established that in the patients that had a good response to spinal adjustment there was a definite rise in the blood glucose level, while at the other end of the swing we found that patients showing little or no response to spinal adjustment showed no change in blood glucose level, and these were mostly cases that had resisted all the usual kinds of treatment and carried a doubtful prognosis.

"It would, of course, be impracticable to give details of the actual laboratory techniques used in making these tests in this work, but the hope was expressed that opportunity of demonstrating this technique to colleagues in the near future was possible.

"All I can do here is to mention that Dr. Dee used the colorimetric method for 'true sugar' in 0·05 ml. of blood."

I was privileged to see some of these tests carried out at the surgery of *Parnell Bradbury*, and I would like to convey my thanks and admiration to these men for their contribution to our science.

CHAPTER THIRTEEN

A Summary by the Author

I feel that some type of summary is necessary at this point in view of the fact that much of the material contained within this book will be subject to some criticism and much controversy, especially in Europe, where the science is just beginning to manifest itself.

The first and all subsequent colleges of chiropractice until the year 1965 have been developed in Canada and the United States and at the time of writing they number sixteen. The "approved" or, as we call them, the "Accredited Colleges" are listed by the official national associations, that is the *International Chiropractic Association* (I.C.A.), 741 Brady Street, Davenport, Iowa, U.S.A., to whom any person may write for information about the Science of Chiropractice, its personnel, training requirements, information about any particular college, legal position in various countries; and the *American* Chiropractic Association (A.C.A.).

Any information directly affecting Europeans may be obtained from the Secretary, European Union of Chiropractors, Zuchwilerstrasse 10, 4500 Solothurn, Switzerland. An Anglo-European College of Chiropractice situated at Bournemouth is expected to be opened at the time this book is published.

The twentieth-century re-discovery of the science of chiropractice was the work of the Canadian, *D. D. Palmer in 1895* and its major development was the life effort of his son, *B. J. Palmer, D.C., Ph.C.*, very ably assisted by his wife *Mabel Heath Palmer*, doctor and anatomist, while the present high academic standards to be found at the Palmer Chiropractic College, are the result of the tireless efforts of the grandson of the original D. D. Palmer, one *David D. Palmer, D.C., Ph.C.*, president of the Palmer Chiropractic College since 1961, ably assisted by his fine faculty.

The developer, B. J. Palmer, had to face the ridicule of the layman and professional men alike in his early days, together with legal opposition from those who, through an absence of knowledge of chiropractice, and chiropractors, forced through an ill-timed malpractice act in many of the states. This Act, while it inconvenienced many chiropractors, and deprived many ordinary citizens of their skill, served the most useful purpose possible, by creating publicity, knowledge of the potential uses of spinal adjustments, and the arousing of public indignation at the injustice of the malpractice act, as it applied to doctors of chiropractice and the resultant removal of these "Acts" from the statute books, followed by granting of licences to practise "The Art and Science of Chiropractice".

I would like to affirm, and to add to my own, the opinions of the bulk of my colleagues, that all credit should be shown to the advances made in the medical world, by the scientists, medical doctors, and especially the surgeons, during the last fifty years, while agreeing wholeheartedly, that the use of drugs is often indicated in the early stages of many disabilities, diseases, and accidents. We likewise are of the opinion, that a continuation of them beyond a *reasonable period* should not be undertaken, if a test period of withdrawal of such drugs results in the return of evidences of original discomfort. There is sometimes evidence that in suppressing pain we are concealing what might be a serious threat to life and health, that could progress rapidly unobserved, for pain is nature's way of making us aware of some threat to our well-being, and it behoves us to look for the *cause*, not deaden beyond a *reasonable* time its *expression and effect*.

In publishing writings, observations, translations, and quotations from authoritative medical writings, covering the last thirty to forty years, it is not my wish or intention to decry, deride or disparage, any remarks or statements made by any member of the medical profession, past or present. My purpose has been to show step by step how, over the years, the opinions of many of the leading medical men, have gradually been made aware of the importance of the spinal column in its relation to health. And the opinion of the doctors who have thoroughly researched our activities has changed, first from *open hostility* in the first quarter of the century, truly a case of condemnation without investigation, to an *understanding tolerance* from 1925 to 1950, and in this third quarter of the century to an *acceptance and friendliness* towards the practitioners of our science.

This has reached the point where many medical doctors send their patients, who in their opinion would benefit from spinal manipulation, to our surgeries for attention. What strikes me so forcibly, is the friendliness that exists between so many of the most enlightened of the medical profession and the present day doctors of chiropractice. I am convinced that much of the credit for this state is due to the greatly improved standard of education and instruction at the advanced chiropractic colleges, the high percentage of recoveries of patients in a shorter period of time whose disabilities can, directly, or indirectly, be attributed to spinal imbalance, and the dropping of the idea that chiropractice is a *cure-all; it is not,* neither is any other healing science. They all have their niche to fill in the restoration and maintenance of health in modern man.

The references and data submitted on *Spinal Balance* were written and published by D. L. Leigh Steinbach, D.C., from whom I received the authority to reprint. It is *part* of a well-written instructive book based on the findings of his father, former Dean of the Universal Chiropractic College. While probably not too interesting for the layman, it is of great interest to the professionals (medical, osteopathic, natureopaths and chiropractors).

The Scofield Chiropractic Charity Trust exists for the chronic cases requiring attention, entailing much expenditure of time and money.

They impressed the need, in the mind of the author of this book, for the creation of a charity trust to assist the less fortunate amongst us to obtain Chiropractic Health Service in England. Eventually perhaps, with the addition of hundreds of chiropractic practitioners, graduating from accredited colleges, making available the specialized services for those in need of them throughout the country, it could become possible for services to be obtained via the National Health Service in a similar way that patients benefit from dentists, opticians, and physiotherapists.

It is to the advantage of the patient in particular, and the nation as a whole, that Chiropractic Health Service should be placed high on the list of essential services to the nation. It would lessen the recovery time of those suffering from spinal disorders such as sciatica and lumbago when produced by herniated, or, more popularly known, as slipped disc.

The exact reproduction of the sections of the *Trust Deed* that has been registered, after approval by *Her Majesty's Charity Trust Commissioners, London, England*, and the *Chief Inspector of Taxes*, as it applies to those whom the *Founder* of the Trust *Arthur G. Scofield, D.C.M.B.C.A.*, of Richmond Lodge, Sudbury, Suffolk, England, intended the said trust to benefit, follows.

Feb 15th 1964. Now this deed WITNESSETH as follows

1. *The Public Custodian* has been authorized to act in place of ordinary Trustees and the administration of the Trust has been vested in the Charity Trust Committee, comprising a president, chairman, treasurer, secretary with a total committee membership of sixteen, and as such has been duly accepted and registered. The trustees hereby declare that they, and the survivors or survivor of them, or other trustees or trustee hereof for the time being, will hold all subscriptions, donations, bequests and other moneys and property, as and when the same shall be paid or vested in them to be held upon the trusts of this deed and the moneys, investments and property from time to time representing the same upon trust to apply the same in accordance with the provisions hereinafter contained to relieve poverty and sickness among poor persons by any or all of the following means:

   A. The making of grants, loans, or contributions towards the cost of obtaining X-ray Photographs before treatment by a chiropractor.
   B. The payment of a chiropractor's fees for treatment.
   C. The provisions, equipment and maintenance of clinics.
   D. The making of contributions to patients who are unable to afford to pay the expense of travelling to and from clinics.
   E. The making of grants, loans, or contributions and the expenditure of money to enable the service of chiropractors to be made available to persons who would otherwise be unable to pay for such services.

F. The making of grants or loans towards the cost of training chiropractors.

2. The name of the Charity shall be *The Scofield Chiropractic Charity Trust.*

The British Chiropractic Laymen's Fellowship (East Anglian Branch) was formed several years ago, following on the pattern first created in England by Doctors Donald and Elizabeth Bennett, D.C.s, of Guildford, Surrey. While some additions to the aims have been made by the *East Anglian Branch*, whose central office is at Richmond Lodge, Sudbury, Suffolk, England, the principle remains that:

The British Chiropractor's Association has long realized the necessity for a LAYMEN's Fellowship to sponsor the requirements of the public for the services of Doctors of Chiropractic in England, and therefore the East Anglian Branch of the Fellowship laid down the following as being applicable in Great Britain, and the aims of such a fellowship would be to:

1. Protect the interests of the public in matters relating to chiropractic care through necessary legislation to recognize the worthiness of the profession and its service to the community.

2. To make the necessary representation to benevolent societies, clubs and health insurance groups, to enable you to obtain the benefits to which you are entitled from any of these when you are temporarily disabled through accidents and strains, which prevent you from attending to your business or place of employment. (*Few of the policies you now hold make provision for chiropractic care* so often necessary for quick recovery.) There are over five hundred insurance groups, benevolent societies and clubs plus workman's compensation clubs in the United States and Canada that carry a clause entitling their members to claim benefits under the signature of their local doctor of chiropractic.

3. To make scholarships available at accredited Colleges of Chiropractice to assist young men and women to become graduate "Doctors of Chiropractice". These would be allocated from the surplus membership funds, as and when available.

4. To educate its members into the care and attention (so necessary to health) of that wonderful, but often uncared for body of yours, through frequent lectures by authoritative teachers.

5. To assist the newly graduated doctors of chiropractice to get established quickly in their new localities.

In 1965 there was formed in Great Britain a new group with which we are affiliated, named the *British Pro-Chiropractic Association* under the able chairmanship of *Sir Frank Markham, M.A., B.Litt.*, which is another step forward towards securing insurance coverage, and Parliamentary action to secure ultimate acceptance within the National Health Service, since this organization is securing members from all parts of the country and we intend giving them all our support.

The Chiropractic Advancement Association (originally entitled *The British Pro-Chiropractic Association* and founded in 1965) is an independent voluntary organization of chiropractic patients who, because of their satisfaction with chiropractic diagnostic and treatment methods for dealing with spinal and pelvic defects and the neurological problems that flow from these, decided to form the Association with the objects of

1. Publicizing chiropractic therapy to enable more to become aware of its benefits.
2. Ensuring that the therapy continued to be available in the United Kingdom to sufferers with musculo-skeletal complaints.
3. Making representations to the Health Authorities on the extended use of chiropractic care in the public interest.
4. Assisting the Anglo-European College of Chiropractic at Bournemouth to provide the best possible facilities for the training of chiropractors wishing to practise in the United Kingdom.

The Association can claim some success in this work. Much remains to be done, the progress of which depends largely on the support available from patients and ex-patients. It has a distinguished Panel of Patrons headed by the President, Dame Janet Baker D.B.E.

Communications to the Secretary, 38 The Island, Thames Ditton, Surrey KT7 0SQ. (Telephone 01-398 2098). Publications: *The British Chiropractic Handbook.*

CHAPTER FOURTEEN

List of Accredited Chiropractic Colleges

EXAMPLES OF TRAINING

Many people are interested in the training and educational background of the modern doctor of chiropractic, and some will be giving thought to the possibility of taking it up as a career. Therefore, I hope the information contained in this chapter will be of particular assistance to them.

In North America, where the first chiropractic college was established in 1895 by the discoverer of the chiropractic principle, Daniel David Palmer, there are now 14 more chiropractic educational colleges. Thousands of doctors of chiropractic have graduated from these first-professional degree granting institutions, and have provided health care for millions of patients. Thus, the merits of the science are well understood and accepted. Licences to practice are granted only to those passing the necessary examinations laid down to comply with the state laws.

In the European world, however, only Switzerland has a system of licence for doctors of chiropractic on a similar basis. However, as more and more chiropractors establish themselves in Europe, other countries will quickly follow. It is natural, therefore, that the laymen of Europe wish to know in reasonable detail the particulars of the education and training doctors of chiropractic have received. With this in mind, I have selected two colleges as examples. Both colleges subscribe to the policies and regulations of the Council on Chiropractic Education, and the C.C.E. Commission on Accreditation, which is recognized by the United States Commission on Accreditation.

The two chosen were selected because of personal knowledge through graduation, frequent postgraduate seminars and the author's place of original practice before pioneering in Europe. They are the **Palmer College** of Chiropractic, the first chiropractic college, which was established late in the last century, and the Canadian Memorial Chiropractic College.

At the Palmer College no student can graduate until he has completed a minimum classroom attendance of 4,320 hours. The student must also satisfy the Dean and Faculty of his proficiency by passing the examinations laid down and fulfilling other specified requirements. Then, providing there is nothing unprofessional in his conduct, the student will graduate as a doctor of chiropractic and will receive a diploma attesting to this.

The term chiropractic, chiropractor or D.C. after his name is essential in display so the science will be distinctive and not confused with medicine.

The principal subject matter of training is outlined in the following list, and while for the sake of saving space, lecture and practical hours are grouped together, the exact differentials may be obtained either from the college bulletin or by writing directly to Palmer College.

Chiropractic Philosophy	180 hours
Anatomy (Myology, Osteology, Histology, Embryology, Introduction to Chirpractic Science, Splanchnology, Genesiology/Angiology, Central Nuerology, Peripheral Neurology, Dissection, Special Senses, Clinical Anatomy)	672
Physiology (Control Systems, Cell Physiology, Digestion/ Nutrition, Endocrinology, Nuerophysiology, Cardiovascular, Renal and Pulmonary, Correlative Physiology Lab)	468
Chemistry (Organic, Biochemistry, Chemistry Lab, Physiological Chemistry and	

Toxicology)	360
Pathology, (Microbiology, Hematology, General Pathology, Subluxation Pathology, General Pathology, Public Health and Sanutation, Cardiovascular Pathology, Gastrointestinal Pathology, Urogenital Pathology)	600
Chiropractic Technique (Technique-Roentgenology I, II, III, IV, V, VI, Technique Review)	400
Roentgenology (Technique-Roentgenology I, II, III, IV, V, VI, Physics, Positioning, Diagnosis-Roentgenology I, II, III, Roentgenology Review)	452
Diagnosis (Physical Diagnosis Method, Diagnosis-	

Roentgenology I, II, III,	Behavior, Geriatrics)	672
Obstetrics and	Clinic (Clinic I, II, III, IV, V,	
Gynecology, Pediatrics	Ethics and Jurisprudence,	
and Febrile Disorders,	Correlative Diagnosis)	516
Diagnosis, Dynamics of		

TOTAL: 4,320 hours

The students of the Palmer College of Chiropractic together with those of other recognized colleges are, therefore, well trained, as indeed they must be to pass the necessary examinations for qualifications for a State Licence to practice.

The four-academic-year course of study at a chiropractic college must be preceded by two years of pre-professional education at college level with emphasis on the sciences.

The chiropractic profession, like those others caring for the health of mankind, has its own associations in the individual states, provinces and countries. The International Chiropractors Association, 1901 "L" Street NW, Washington, D.C. 20036, U.S.A., is willing to assist your enquiries about the profession and can readily state whether the particular college of your choice is an accredited one.

The curriculum at P.C.C. is structured in two parts – basic science and clinical science. The basic sciences include anatomy with individual and general labs, chemistry with clinical chemistry lab, physiology and pathology. The clinical sciences include x-ray, technique, diagnosis, clinic and philosophy.

Theory courses in the various anatomies place heavy emphasis on the nervous system and its relation to chiropractic. Lecture courses in myology, osteology, splanchnology, angiology, genesiology, nuerology, special senses and spinal anatomy are complemented by detailed labs in these areas. A general laboratory experience in human dissection culminates the almost two academic years of anatomical study.

Students arrive at P.C.C. having completed pre-chiropractic liberal arts studies in inorganic and organic chemistry. The chemistry courses taught, therefore, are those specifically related to the human organism, vis: biochemistry.

Courses in physiology complement and follow closely the anatomy curriculum. A physiology lab is utilized to give the student practical experience in the various physiological mechanisms of the human body. Once the student is schooled in the anatomy and physiology of the body, he is assisted in identifying anatomical and physiological abnormalities through corresponding courses in pathology.

In the clinical science area Palmer students are given instruction in the science and art of chiropractic. Courses include technique, x-ray, diagnosis and clinic.

The technique package gives the student a broad base of chiropractic methodology. The x-ray department prepares students in the method and diagnosis of roentgenological films. Diagnosis courses lead the student in a path to the identification of disease and abnormal physiology.

The clinic at Palmer College begins the active practice of each student. It is in the Clinic that the student learns while under the watchful eye of skilled chiropractors on the staff, how to treat patients as whole human beings. Rigorous requirements for graduation ensure a high degree of clinical competency.

The philosophy programme at Palmer College is second to none in the chiropractic world. Each student is carefully guided through the history and philosophy of the profession in courses which are strategically placed throughout the academic calendar.

The physical plant at Palmer College in the past few years has been extensively remodelled and developed to provide the most modern clinical setting in the profession today.

BASIC PRINCIPLES TAUGHT BY CANADIAN MEMORIAL CHIROPRACTIC COLLEGE

The Canadian Memorial Chiropractic College states that National Examining Boards have been established (by the Chiropractic Profession) in both Canada and the United States, with the approval and assistance of universities in both countries. Licensing Boards of Provincial and State Governments are accepting the national examinations. This development was initiated by the Canadian Chiropractic Association through its Committee on Education, which has worked for eight years to establish its National Examining Board. In Canada, national examinations were commenced in 1963. In the United States they were held for the first time in 1965. This development will help to maintain uniform professional standards across Canada and successful candidates may apply for licensure in the various provinces.

Chiropractic College Course of Study. Your modern chiropractor completes a college course which is equivalent in hours to a five-year university course, but which is condensed into four years at the Canadian Memorial Chiropractic College. This is accomplished by requiring the students to attend classes for nine months during the year instead of seven.

Basic science forms an important part of the chiropractic curriculum which includes the following subjects: Anatomy (including human dissection), Chemistry, Bacteriology, Physiology, Pathology, Diagnosis, Roentgenology, Paediatrics, Psychology, Obstetrics, Gynaecology, Jurisprudence, Chiropractic principles and techniques, Public Health, etc., etc.

Clinic Internship is added to the normal lecture hours during the last three semesters of the course, thus increasing the load upon the student, but presenting him with the opportunity of applying the knowledge he has gained. One of his most important responsibilities is to determine which patients require chiropractic care and which should seek the services of other practitioners. The modern chiropractor is trained to recognize the patient's needs in this respect and to refer him for other types of care as required.

CONTENT OF THE COURSE

Matriculation requirements for the Canadian Memorial Chiropractic College have always been High School graduation, good morals, character, and health. In recent years the entrance requirements have been increased to "the educational standing required for entrance to a university or similar institute of higher learning" or Ontario Secondary School Honour Graduation for this province. A number of students have had some university education and a percentage have academic degrees.

The course is divided into four academic years of nine months each with each year consisting of two semesters of 18 weeks each. The subjects and hours, as listed, have been followed with precision and it will be noted that the first two years are concerned primarily with the basic science subjects that form the foundation of any education in healing. During the third year greater emphasis is given the clinical subjects, which are continued into the fourth year, to be supplemented by speciality subjects, such as paediatrics, abnormal psychology, etc.

The student of chiropractice has a required schedule of thirty lecture and laboratory hours per week. In his third year he is required to serve additional hours in clinic; first caring for the needs of fellow students under close supervision of the staff, then assisting in the laboratories of the out-patient clinic and serving in the capacity of observer-clerk for senior internes. After passing practical examination and oral questionings of the clinic staff, he is admitted as an interne with the privilege of accepting patients to be diagnosed and treated under supervision.

A comparison of hours devoted by chiropractic and medical students to master the same subjects is found favourable in chiropractic; as illustrated later in this brief. Gross developmental and microscopic anatomy are thoroughly taught by means of lectures, projected illustrations, small animal dissection, microscopic studies in embryology and histology. After completion of the study of gross anatomy in systematic form, the student reviews the entire subject by the regional method of dissection of the human cadaver. Cadavers are supplied by the General Inspector of Anatomy for the Province of Ontario. In all, 900 hours are devoted to every phase of anatomy, supplemented by the surface anatomy studies provided in the department of chiropractic technique.

Physiology occupies 342 hours of the course with every phase of normal function receiving consideration. The class room instruction is supported by experimentation in the laboratory.

Chemistry occupies a portion of three semesters for a total of 306 hours in instruction and laboratory application. Inorganic and organic chemistry courses provide the basis for the detailed consideration of physiology or Bio-Chemistry, which is of greater practical importance to the understanding of human function in health or disease.

A part of each of four semesters is devoted to the subject of Pathology for a total of 414 hours, covering the gamut of tissue change in disease.

Bacteriology, Hygiene, and Public Health receive consideration in 270 hours of instructions, laboratory study, and field trips. The Doctor of Chiropractice must be familiar with the collection of micro-organisms, their culture, mounting on slides, staining and identification under a microscope. He must be acquainted with the accepted methods employed for good hygiene and sanitation, as well as being well informed on the laws governing infectious and contagious diseases and other public health problems. He is equipped to render an intelligent advisory service in his community and to co-operate intelligently with the local Department of Public Health.

Both Normal and Abnormal Psychology provide the student with an understanding of the functioning of the human mind and the knowledge to diagnose the deviations from normal with emphasis upon the signs and symptoms indicative of the need for the specialist or institutionalization of the patient. These courses require 108 hours.

Diagnosis requires 342 hours of study to encompass case history technique, subjective and objective symptoms, and physical examination; 108 hours of instruction in laboratory investigation as a source of diagnostic information includes urinalysis, blood counts, sedimentation rate, blood analysis, bacterial smears, gastric and foecal analysis, etc., and the specialized instrumentation such as electrocardiography, endocardiography, basal metabolism assessment, and audiometric investigations. Still another 144 hours are occupied with the speciality subjects of Dermatology, Ophthalmology, Oto-Laryngology, and Paediatrics.

Obstetrics and Gynaecology with the care of expectant mothers, the signs and symptoms of complication in the natural process of pregnancy and post-partal care is taught in 108 hours of instruction.

The consideration of x-rays occupies 198 classrooms and laboratory hours to familiarize the student with the physics of x-ray, the indications, contra-indications, hazards, protective devices, and techniques, as well as the technique of taking quality radiographs of the spine and the entire osseous structures. Considerable time is devoted to the analysis of structural distortion and the recognition of pathological change as exemplified by the radiographic films.

In addition to the didactic study each student must spend a minimum of three weeks internship in the x-ray department, applying his knowledge of roentgenology procedure and during his clinic internship is required to be present for the x-ray examination of each of his patients; then to read the roentgenograms and write the report of his findings for examination by the head of the department and the Clinic Director. The Commission should bear in mind that in the application of the roentgen-ray the chiropractor never uses it for treatment, nor does he undertake such specialized studies as would require the introduction of foreign substances into the cavities of the body or contrast media given by hypodermic injection. Many cases are referred to competent radiologists for these specialized investigations and many roentgenograms are forwarded for expert interpretation once the pathological process has been observed.

756 hours are devoted to the principles, philosophy, methods of structural analysis, instruments for detection of the sites of nerve interference, and the techniques of chiropractice for the care of the sick and suffering. In addition, the student must spend a minimum of 540 hours of practical application of his basic science knowledge, diagnostic skill, and treatment art, to the handling of sick people in the ambulatory clinic of the college.

Dietetics, Office Management, Chiropractic Jurisprudence, Board Review, First Aid and Emergency Treatment, account for another 270 hours to provide a grand total of 4,806 hours of intensive learning prior to qualifying as a Doctor of Chiropractice (D.C.).

An optional course is offered in Drugless Therapy, taught in the afternoons and evenings after the regular class schedule, to provide for those desirous of acquiring the knowledge of the indications, contra-indications, and techniques of application of adjunctive measures, such as exercise, electro-therapy, etc. This course provides knowledge and experience necesssary for the application by the chiropractor of these measures, or the assessment of the needs of the patient and the intelligent prescription of treatment by a physiotherapist or occupational therapist.

We have now described in brief form the educational experience to which the chiropractic student is exposed and must successfully complete prior to graduation. The following table is submitted to illustrate the comparison of similar studies taken by students, leading to the degree of Doctor of Medicine or Chiropractice. These figures have been taken from the respective 1960–61 calendars of the two colleges of the University of Toronto and that of the Canadian Memorial Chiropractic College. Of necessity, the aforementioned subjects have required a modified grouping for comparison purposes, and any disparity in presentation is apparent and not absolute.

COMPARISON OF TEACHING HOURS
as indicated in the 1960–61 calendars of each college

SUBJECTS		MEDICINE University of Toronto	CHIROPRACTICE Canadian Memorial Chiropractic College
Anatomy:			
Gross		268	612
Microscopic		138	108
Comparative		180 (pre)★	
Developmental			126
	TOTAL	586	900
Chemistry		534 (320 pre)★	306
Professional		522	936
Clinic		623	540
Bacteriology		?	180
Physiology		235	342
English		84 (pre)★	20 (optional)
Public Health		136	90
Diagnosis		427 (plus clinic)	462 (plus clinic)
First Aid		?	36
Pathology		?	414
X-ray		25	198
Jurisprudence		10 (plus)	54
Psychology		?	
Obs. and Gyn.		76	108
Paediatrics		48 (plus clinic)	54 (plus clinic)
Pathologic Chem.		156	108
Physical Med.		16	180 (optional)

★ Preprofessional course.

From this comparison it should be appreciated that the chiropractic student is well equipped by didactic presentation to stand in the light of equality with the graduates of medicine of the University of Toronto. Of course, it must be realized that the benefits of hospitals, and the more extended course in the humanities, represent a distinct advantage to the medical student.

FINAL SCHEDULE FOR 1965–66

FIRST SEMESTER

Subject	Material	Lecture	Lab.	Total	Hours per week
Anatomy I	Osteology and Arthrology	72			
Histology		63	27		
Orthopedy		36			
Physiology	Protoplasm and Cells	72	18		
Chemistry I	General	54	36		
Philosophy I		36			
Orientation and Tech.	Intro. to Palpation	18	18		
		351	99	450	25

SECOND SEMESTER

Anatomy II	Myology	72			
Anatomy III	Splanchnology	72			
Embryology		72			
Chemistry II	Organic	72	36		
Technique II	Palpation		54		
First Aid			36		
X-ray I		18	36		
		306	162	468	26

THIRD SEMESTER

Anatomy IV	Central Nervous System	72			
Physiology II	Muscle and Nerve Cells	18			
Chemistry III	Bio-chemistry	72	36		
Pathology I	Introduction	72			
Bacteriology I	Intro-Parasitology	54			
Diagnosis I	Viral etc.	54			
Philosophy II		36			
Technique IIIa	Stance—Leverage		36		
Technique IIIb	Cleavage		18		
		378	90	468	26

FOURTH SEMESTER

Anatomy V	Peripheral Nervous S.	90			
Physiology III	Metabolism-Endocrinology	72			
Pathology II	Specific Organs	72	36		
Bacteriology II	Classification-Lab-Mycology	54	72		
Diagnosis II	Chem. Agents, etc.	72			
Technique IVa	Stance and Leverage		18		
Technique IVb	Cleavage		36		
		360	162	522	29

FIFTH SEMESTER

Anatomy VI	Angiology	90			
Physiology IVa	Special senses	18			
Physiology IVb	Nervous system	54			
Physiology IVc	Respiration—Cardiac	54			
Diagnosis III	Genito-Urinary, etc.	72		(630 hours	
Lab. Diagnosis		36	36	w/clinic)	
X-ray II	Spinal column	18	36		
Technique Va	Accessory		36		
Technique Vb	Reflex		18		
Ch. Instrumentation			54		
Clinic				108 (6 hrs.	
				w/wk)	
		342	180	522	29

SIXTH SEMESTER

Anatomy VII	Dissection		108		
Nutritional Hygiene		36			
Pathology III	Specific organs	72	36		
Orthopaedics			54		(666 hours
Professional Ec.		54			w/clinic)
x-ray III	Diagnostic	54			
Philosophy III		36			
Technique VIa	Reflex—30		30		
Technique VIb	Leverage—12		12		
Technique VIc	Cleavage—12		12		
Clinic					216 (12 hrs/ wk)
		252	252	504	28

SEVENTH SEMESTER

Pathology IV	Special and Dental	54	18		
Clinic Diag.: Seminar			36		
Jurisprudence		36			
San. and Public health		54	36		(864 hours
Gynaecology and Obstetrics		72			w/clinic)
Normal Psychology		54			
X-ray IV	Soft tissue—Legal reports	54			
Technique VII	Correlation		36		
Clinic					396 (22 hrs/ wk)
		324	126	450	25

EIGHTH SEMESTER

Board Review (Anat. 18) (Path. 18) (X-ray 18) (Chem. 18)	72			
Dermatology	36			
Clinic. Diag. Seminar		36		
E.E.N.T.	54			
Paediatrics	54			(666 hours
Abnormal Psychology	54			w/clinic)
Correl. of Dysfunction and Treatment	54			
Public speaking	18			
Philosophy IV	36			
Technique VIII Correlation		18		
Clinic			216	
	378	54	432	24

TOTALS:	2644	1152	936	4752

THE NATIONAL COLLEGE OF CHIROPRACTIC

200 East Roosevelt Road, Lombard, Illinois 60148
United States of America

This College was originally located in Chicago in 1908 where it was chartered and incorporated under the laws of the State of Illinois, but due to the increasing student body (at present nearly one thousand) it was relocated in 1963 at the above address.

The President of the National College of Chiropractic is Dr Joseph Janse who has held this position for many years. He is an able lecturer, having addressed the Doctors of Chiropractic in many countries, and he is one of the fifteen Doctors of the Council on Chiropractic Education.

The Dean of Admissions and Records of the National College is R.P. Beideman, D.C. from whom information can be obtained about the College, or other accredited colleges named by the Council of Chiropractic Education in the following list taken from the American Chiropractic Association's Journal of Chiropractic of April 1979.

THE COUNCIL ON CHIROPRACTIC EDUCATION

Accredited Status

Los Angeles College of Chiropractic
Dr W. Heath Quigley, President
920 East Broadway
Glendale, CA 91205 (213) 240-7686

National College of Chiropractic
Dr. Joseph Janse, President
200 East Roosevelt Road
Lombard, IL 60148 (312) 629-2000

Northwestern College of Chropractic
Dr. John B. Wolfe, President
1834 S. Mississippi River Blvd
St Paul, MN 55116 (612) 690-1735

Texas Chiropractic College
Dr. John B. Barfoot, President
5912 Spencer Highway
Pasadena, TX 77505 (713) 487-1170

Logan College of Chiropractic
Dr. William N. Coggins, President
1851 Schoettler Road, Box 100
Chesterfield, MO 63017 (314) 227-2100

New York Chiropractic College
Dr. Ernest G. Napolitano, President
Post Office Box 167
Glen Head, NY 11545 (516) 626-2700

Recognized Candidate
for Accreditation Status

Cleveland Chiropractic College
Dr. Carl Cleveland Jr. President
6401 Rockhill Road
Kansas City, MO 64131 (816) 333-8230

Palmer College of Chiropractic
Dr Galen Price, President
1000 Brady Street
Davenport, IA 52830 (319) 324-1611

Western States Chiropractic College
Dr. Richard Timmins, President
2900 NE 132nd Avenue
Portland, OR 97230 (503) 256-3180

Correspondent Status

Life Chiropractic College
Dr. Sid Williams, President
1269 Barclay Circle, Suite A
Marietta, GA 30062 (404) 425-0554

Other Member Colleges

Cleveland Chiropractic College
Dr Carl Cleveland Sr. President
590 North Vermont Avenue
Los Angeles, CA 90004 (213) 660-6166

Pasadena College of Chiropractic
Dr. Arthur Garrow, President
55 North St John Avenue
Pasadena, CA 91101 (213) 449-2466

Northern California College of Chiropractic
Dr. Thomas A. Vonder Haar, President
655 Arastradero Road
Palo Alto, CA 94306 (415) 493-8836

Affiliate Member Colleges

Canadian Memorial Chiropractic College
Dr. D.C. Sutherland, President
1900 Bayview Avenue
Toronto 17, Ontario
Canada (416) 482-2340

International College of Chiropractic
Dr. Andres M. Kleynhans, Principal
Post Office Box 96
Bundoora VIC 3083
Australia

Anglo-European College of Chiropractic
Dr. A. Christensen, Dean
Cavendish Road, Bournemouth
England, BH1 1RA Bournemouth 24777

There are twelve laboratories in the National College, which are designed for class teaching as well as research, with which are associated Departmental Offices.

Laboratory instruction is provided in the following disciplines: Biomechanics, Chemistry, Chiropractice, Diagnosis, Anatomy, Microbiology, Pathology, Physiological Therapeutics, Physiology, Roentgenology, and Clinical Practice

The National College of Chiropractic is a five year co-educational, private professional, non-profit making Academic institution (in 1968 the two-year pre-professional requirement for admission became effective).

INTERNATIONAL CHIROPRACTORS ASSOCIATION

Solely responsible for University of Colorado Chiropractic research project.

Responsible for $2 million appropriation from Congress for chiropractic research.

Responsible, therefore, for the NINDS Conference in February 1975.

ICA/University of Colorado received first federal money for chiropractic research.

University of Colorado has developed computer-aided X-ray analysis and first basic research evident that spinal nerve roots are 'exquisitely' sensitive to pressure.

University of Colorado has developed the most sophisticated computer programme in history on the three-dimensional dynamic spine. The automotive industry has recently purchased this programme to use in the simulation of auto accidents and resultant injury to spinal structures. A film on this will be available soon from the ICA.

FACTS – Foundation for the Advancement of Chiropractic Tenets and Science, a foundation formed by the ICA has won the first HEW contract ever awarded for a study of the costs of chiropractic education, the demand for chiropractic services and the cost of such services. This study is on-going.

The ICA is sponsoring the first International Scientific

Conference on the Spine – sponsored by a chiropractic organization – scheduled for Anaheim, California in late February. M.D.'s, D.C.'s and independent scientists are taking part. A major textbook will be published as a result of this Conference.

The ICA is actively supporting – and has been for three years – the anti-trust suit filed in federal court in Chicago, Illinois by five chiropractors against the AMA and fifteen other major defendants. We are optimistic about the outcome.

The ICA's move to Washington, D.C. has already resulted in many favourable accomplishments:

a.   Active work on Medicare,
b.   Inclusion in several Federal Employee Health Benefit Contracts,
c.   Direct communications with HEW, the Civil Service Commission, the Congress and the Medical Sciences Division of the Museum of History and Technology of the Smithsonian Institution.

The ICA has instituted a new publication, mailed monthly, on matters pertaining to the federal government. This publication is already becoming a major professional resource for detailed information on chiropractic in federal legislation. The name of the publication is the *Washington Legislation Today*.

CURRENTLY APPROVED I.C.A. COLLEGES

Cleveland Chiropractic College of Kansas City
6401 Rockhill Road, Kansas City, MO 64131 (816) 333-8230

Cleveland Chiropractic College of Los Angeles
590 North Vermont Avenue, Los Angeles, CA 90004 (213) 660-6166

New York Chiropractic College
P.O. Box 167
Glen Head, New York (516) 626-2700

Life Chiropractic College
1269 Barclay Circle, Marietta, GA 30062 (404) 424-0554

Logan College of Chiropractic
430 Schoettler Rd, P.O. Box 100
Chesterfield, Missouri 63017 (314) 227-2100

Palmer College of Chiropractic
1000 Brady Street, Davenport, Iowa 52803 (319) 324-1611

Sherman College of Chiropractic
P.O. Box 1452, 2020 Springfield Road
Spartanburgn, S.C. 29304 (803) 578-8770

ANGLO-EUROPEAN COLLEGE OF CHIROPRACTIC
Bournemouth, England

The college began its activities in 1965, registered as a non-profit charitable organization. A second building was purchased in the following year, thus permitting a much needed expansion of laboratory and clinic facilities.

The educational policy of the college is to provide the best possible education and training in the basic and clinical sciences to students wanting to enter the Chiropractic profession. Also to provide post-graduate courses for field practitioners and to establish a research centre.

The teaching is geared not only to impart the scientific facts, but also the ability to utilize them in the prevention and treatment of pain, illness, and disease. The college also endeavours to impart an awareness of the prestige and responsibility a professional person carries as a result of the knowledge obtained, and to develop a sense of maturity and need for professional, civic, and moral ethics.

Emphasis is placed on the scientific soundness of Chiropractic principles and effectiveness of the Chiropractic treatment covering all phases of spinal adjustment, manipulative techniques and related measures.

Admission requirements: Students must be at least seventeen years of age. No discrimination as to sex, race, or religion. English being the language of instruction, all students must be proficient in this language.

In Britain: Three passes at 'Advanced' level to include Biology or Zoology and Chemistry.

Scotland: Four passes in S.C.E. 'Highers' with a minimum of 'B' pass, to include Biology or Zoology and Chemistry.

British Commonwealth: University entrance or equivalent in Biology or Zoology and Chemistry.

U.S.A. and Canada: Two years in an accredited junior college, college or university, to include Biology or Zoology and Chemistry.

Mature age candidates: Any person over 23 years of age may apply under the mature age provision.

The course is a four year, full-time study totalling over 4,500 hours including a twelve month period of clinic internship amounting to 1,000 hours, leading to a Diploma of 'Doctor of Chiropractic' and a Diploma of 'Roentgenology'.

In addition to the final written examinations, each student must complete a project/thesis and pass the final Clinical Proficiency Examination, which is both viva voce and practical.

Governing Bodies:

Board of Governors – composed of a national representative of each member country of the European Chiropractors' Union.

Board of Regents – responsible for the overall running of the college.

Academic Board.

Faculty Council and its Committees.

The Anglo-European College of Chiropractic is the only training centre for Chiropractic in Europe.

The Science of Health

By Henry J. Langner, D.C., Geneva (Switzerland)

Almost every day the propaganda apparatus of medicine and the pharmaceutical industries announces some sensational progress in the science of medicine. If this so-called progress were real, all people should by now be in excellent health and the sick an exception. In reality more people are sick, or at least in bad health, and every year new and greater hospitals have to be built. The increase of the population and the greater longevity are not sufficient to account for it, since the proportion between the number of the sick and the total population has increased by 40% during the last twenty years.

The well-known philosopher Aldous Huxley said: "Medicine has made such enormous progress, that there are practically no more people in good health."

During the Middle Ages, Europe has known terrific epidemics which in certain places within a few weeks killed more than half of the population. Medicine was absolutely helpless against them because it did not know the causes. Today, we know that an absolute lack of public and personal hygiene were the main causes and that with the introduction of cleanliness and measures like running water in the houses, baths and street cleaning, diseases like pest and cholera have entirely disappeared in civilized countries.

Today the picture has changed but the problem is similar. Again we have illnesses which are fatal to millions of people, like cancer or heart diseases against which medicine is practically as helpless as it was in old times against certain epidemics. The reason is again that medicine doesn't know the causes. People continue to die of cancer by the thousands. For example; in France twenty years ago there was a death from cancer every ten minutes; today it kills a man every five minutes. This in spite of the fact that since about a century ago, millions and millions of dollars have been spent in cancer research. So far with no result.

Many people outside official medicine know that cancer, coronary thrombosis, rheumatism, diabetes and many others, are *diseases of civilization*, caused first by wrong living and eating habits of modern man, second by erroneous medical treatment. In order to win the battle against diseases of civilization *it is necessary to propagate a new hygiene and educate people to live in accordance with the laws of health*.

Pierre Delbet, a French specialist in cancer research, wrote: "It is just as easy to prevent cancer, as it is impossible to cure it. The same is true of the other diseases of civilization."

The majority of people in the Western world have been conditioned to think that a disease is due to bad luck, germs, fate or an imperfection of our bodies. This is not true; most illnesses and *all diseases of civilization are due to errors in our living habits*. To continue these errors and to think that it is enough to swallow some drugs to recover health is a dangerous illusion, which profits only the pharmaceutical industry. Just a few examples of how this illusion is widespread. In the U.S. annually seven million kilos of aspirin are consumed. We have about 6,000 sorts of tranquillizers. For one of them 35 million prescriptions have been delivered during one year. The people of France consume *every day four hundred tons of drugs*. Similar quantities are used in all other civilized countries. The pharmaceutical industries have developed thousands of drugs against all kinds of diseases, even to *the point where drugs have become one of the major causes of disease*. If one considers that there are about 150,000 different drugs on the market, it is permissible to doubt of their efficiency. How is it that primitive races, untouched by civilization, medicine and the drug industry remain healthy without any effort, while in civilized countries more and more people are in bad health?

Today most people's views on health are warped by the absolutely unwarranted preponderance of one therapeutical method which has succeeded in assuming an official position and to become practically a state institution. Thus only the most orthodox medicine is taught in our Universities and this teaching claims to be infallible and established once and for ever.

In order to maintain this usurped reputation of infallibility as well as its monopoly, medicine dispenses a well organized propaganda apparatus. Thus all other methods of healing are systematically discarded.

Medicine is based on a totally wrong concept.

Medicine is based on materialistic theories and hypotheses out of accord with real human nature, which is a living wholeness made of material and immaterial components intricately interwoven. The invisible life forces, the metaphysical part of man which governs the material body, cannot be grasped by means of our present scientific methods. This does not mean that these forces do not exist.

Disease can be defined as the consequences of a disturbance of the human personality, considered as a living wholeness, due to non-observation of the natural laws to which this wholeness is submitted. In other words, disease is an abnormal state of the human organism caused by errors in its living habits. It can also be defined as a reaction of the organism to restore health and order and is accompanied by the appearance of germs, erroneously termed noxious, whereas in reality these are a consequence and not a cause of disease and their mission is precisely to eliminate individuals who live contrary to the law of Nature. This is why medicine with all its more and more powerful chemical "bug hunting" is working against the efforts of nature to restore order. *That is why in the end medicine will be the loser*, and why we have more and more diseases, for the wisdom of the body and of nature is immensely greater than the wisdom of human reason.

To trust this higher order of nature means to use the infinite wisdom of creation out of which man himself came.

It is curious to note that the great majority of medical doctors do not seem to be aware that their methods of treatment are not restoring true health.

If by administrating a drug, an M.D. causes a symptom to disappear, he calls it a cure, or at least a successful treatment, even if *after some time* one discovers that certain organs have been damaged in the process.

He doesn't seem to realize that the passive removal of bothersome symptoms is an error and is at the origin of chronic disease.

After a resection of the stomach the patient is usually not

taught how and what he should eat to avoid a recurrence and is allowed to continue to smoke. But by checking a disease by the use of drugs, the patient is allowed to escape the consequences of his errors and to continue to transgress fundamental laws of nature. Thus the patient is dispensed from *reflecting on the deeper causes of his illness*, and has learned nothing from the experience.

It was *Hippocrates* who has said, "When one has fallen sick we must change our way of living, for it is evident that the one we followed was erroneous wholly or in great part." "It is nature which cures disease, the physician must learn from nature."

This advice is still valid, for natural laws governing the human body are as immutable as those of the planets moving around the sun, contrary to most scientific dogmas which are the *truth of today*, but the *errors of yesterday* and *of tomorrow*.

Official medicine doesn't know the true cause of disease, what *actually happens when a sick person gets well* is unknown to medical science.

It is really amazing that we should have all this confusion, ignorance, make-believe, and false pretense in today's scientific world, and not even seem to realize it, because *commercialism and high pressure salesmanship have an interest to hide the real situation*. Most people do not even care any more to know the truth and are happy to believe what a guileful propaganda tells them about *the wonderful progress of our time*.

There is also a widespread misuse of the word "Health" itself. One talks of World *Health* Organization, Ministry of *Health*, National *Health* Service, etc. Actually these institutions are mainly interested in disease and do not know what real health is and how it can be maintained. Science has not studied the laws of Nature which would permit man to stay in good health without taking any drug at all. The graduates of our medical schools do not have the least inkling of these laws.

It is not my intention to minimize the immense research work done by medical men. The number of scientific periodicals and medical journals is impressive and has increased to a point where even the specialist is no longer able to read all that is written on his own speciality. For instance, in Germany alone there exist 328 scientific medical periodicals covering some sixty specialities. In 1957, there were published the world over 4,358 medical periodicals. In 1956, the manual of internal medicine was published in four volumes, comprising 4,040 pages on diseases of the lungs and bronchi only.

Unfortunately this immense work deals practically only with diseases. A humorous writer wrote in this connection: "It is fortunate that infants can't read because if they could, science would have written a lot of books on the art of suckling and the poor babes would not know how to go about it."

On the other hand, scientists have not written a single manual dealing systematically with health and the laws governing it.

Nobody can deny that official medicine has obtained remarkable results in acute disease with certain life saving drugs. However, this success was obtained in a comparatively small section of medicine, i.e., infectious diseases. Today the main problem, which is that of the chronic degenerative diseases of civilization, has not only remained unsolved but is getting worse, because medicine's methods of treating acute diseases are absolutely inadequate to cope with these chronic diseases which account for by far the greater majority of medicine's patients.

It is necessary to change our way of thinking. Instead of thinking exclusively in terms of diseases, studying disease and searching for ways and means to fight them, we must change and *think in terms of health*, study its laws and find ways and means to have it and keep it. We will then find that it is possible to comprehend health and disease in a way entirely different from that of official science, a way that is much closer to Nature and to common sense; it implies thinking in terms of wholeness.

Health is a state of order resulting from the observation of natural law, while *there is only one state of order* the possibilities of disorder are unlimited and therefore the diseases are countless. Consequently it would be comparatively simple to study and know the laws of health, rather than try and know the countless number of diseases. Nevertheless this is what medicine tries to do. This explains the avalanche of research and writings with no hope of ever coming to an end.

PART TWO

1. The principles of the Science of Health are natural laws, the working of which each one can experience upon himself. All

nature lives according to Universal law. Man being a part of nature has already evolved in accordance with them, must submit to them in order to stay healthy.

2. The Science of Health teaches that the human organism is able to be in perfect health if the laws of his life community are obeyed.

3. Disease is not accidental or just bad luck, but due to transgression of the laws of health. It is just an attempt of living forces to restore health. The Science of Health studies the reasons why disease exists.

4. Nature seeks to eliminate those who do not conform to its laws and disease is a means of elimination.

5. Even germs which wrongly are considered "Pathogenic" are a means of nature to eliminate unhealthiness and disorder. The great majority of germs are useful and absolutely necessary to maintain health.

6. *Health* is not only the absence of disease, but something positive, a state of *exuberant vitality and resistance, a complete and perfect functioning of all organs, practically inexhaustible reserves. Immunity against all infection. Harmony and balance of the whole personality on all levels.*

7. The Science of Health is not identical with preventative medicine. The latter tries to prevent an illness that threatens, by means of early diagnosis and artificial defence, while the former studies and applies the laws of life which permit one to stay in absolute good health. The difference is the same as that between vaccination and the building up of a natural immunity and resistance of the body by healthy living.

8. The Science of Health does not fight any particular germ of disease. Obedience to the laws of life gives our body the possibility to defend itself efficiently against all. The Science of Health is not fighting *against* something, but *for* a normal functioning of the cells and organs, *for* a healthy organic terrain.

9. The Science of Health does not consider the symptoms of disease as something negative that has to be fought at all costs, but considers them as a warning that mistakes have been made and looks for their significance. By eliminating their causes (*mostly transgressions of the laws of life*), they will become useless and disappear by themselves.

10. The Science of Health takes into consideration the invisible life forces which create the material body, animate it, move it, nourish it, and heal it. These forces are also part of the wholeness of the human being and of all living organisms.

11. The Science of Health is not primarily concerned with disease, or early diagnosis of disease, but with the health forces of human organism, in view of their activation, development, and strengthening, in order to allow health to exist and to render disease unnecessary.

12. The Science of Health promotes the health education of man from the beginning, in order to obtain the best possible development of all his natural predispositions and endowments, Physical, Mental, Ethical and Spiritual.

13. The law of life can be explored, observed and described with the same scientific rigour as any other matter, by means of the science of wholeness.

14. The modern hygienist or health educator is neither a M.D. nor a healer, but a biologist in the true sense of the term, a man who discards official and mostly erroneous dogmas and is searching with an open mind and unbiased knowledge of life, for a solution of the most vital problem of a more and more stricken humanity.

15. The Science of Health does not advocate renouncing the advantages of modern technic, but wants to protect man's health against its disadvantages.

16. The Science of Health is therefore in the first place: *Information and teaching of the laws of health*. The public should know that the causes of diseases are infractions of these laws and not something else. The diseases disappear if the laws are obeyed. The Science of Health wants to reawaken the sense of responsibility of every individual for his own health, by supplying all necessary information to do so.

Today we have the most marvellous hospitals, clinics and institutions for the treatment of disease. It would be necessary to have just as perfect establishments to study and promote health. It should be possible to do away with a great number of hospitals and replace them with a great number of educational centres in the art of staying in good health. This should actually be possible, according to a declaration of Dr. Buurmann, Director of public health in the German Federal Republic, at a recent congress of prophylactic medicine. He said that the cost of disease which burdens the national income could be reduced to one per cent of the present amount. How? Simply by teaching people the way of healthy living.

This should be the duty of the State, but the responsible authorities do nothing effectual, because this teaching would render useless the greater part of the M.D. of the Hospitals. *It would ruin the pharmaceutical industries* and those of *alchohol, tobacco* and a *great number of noxious products.* The most formidable interests oppose such a change, because disease and bad health have become one of the most important economic factors.

This means that very profitable business is made with disease and a great number of products which *cause* disease.

This is probably the main reason why nothing changes in spite of all EVIDENCE.

Thus the real problems of health are kept hidden, orchestrated propaganda apparatus continually speaks of progress of medicine, of the creation of miracle drugs and sensational operations, and by doing so the real situation, which is already very alarming, is concealed from the public and people continue to ignore how to stay in good health.

There exist some very fine institutions to help the disabled of all sorts, such as associations for the victims of cancer, diabetes, tuberculosis, multiple sclerosis, rheumatism and many others. All these organizations are to be commended for their fine work to help these unfortunate people, but practically all this misery could be avoided; it is evident that it would be much more rational and less costly, if one would inform all these people since childhood *how to live and stay in good health.*

If the children were instructed in proper living habits, they would develop healthy minds and bodies during the growing age and stay healthy all life long. A proper hygiene should be applied from the first day of life, as the foundation of health is laid during the early development of the child. *If started in the adult age only,* although useful and helpful, these same hygienic measures are not as efficacious any more.

As has already been said, the Science of Health *does not exist yet*, nevertheless certain rules are known and have successfully been put into practice by certain groups of people and a great number of isolated persons, *allowing them to enjoy a state of absolute health*, or to regain health if it has been lost. Here follow some of these rules.

RULES OF HEALTH

1. Man needs adequate, living *unadulterated* food in proper quantities and qualities. Today most civilized men eat food in too great quantity, but deficient in quality and highly toxic.
2. Man needs sufficient movement, effort, and physical exercise to keep all tissues and organs in good form. For instance the strength of the *Cardiac muscles* must be maintained by means of daily efforts, by walking, running, or some exercise. Cardiac weakness due to lack of training is certainly a major cause for the rapid increase in fatal heart disease in recent years. *It is an error to avoid all hardship and difficulty in life* as it makes man weak and defenceless.
3. Man needs good thorough breathing of fresh and pure air in order to secure an abundant supply of oxygen and pure blood to all organs, tissues, and cells.
4. Man must abstain from smoking, drinking in excess spirits, coffee and other stimulants, drugs, etc., these are all detrimental to health.
5. Man needs sufficient rest, relaxation and sleep, natural rhythm between day and night, work and rest, should be observed.
6. Man needs mental, nervous, and emotional stability, Fear, uncontrolled emotions, negative thought patterns, continued nerve tension, noise, etc., are important causes of bad health.
7. Man needs normally functioning and balanced spine and nervous system to stay in good health. Science discovers every day a little more what Chiropractors have known for seventy years, i.e., the importance of good posture for health.
8. Man needs to exercise all his physical, mental, ethical, and spiritual endowments, functions, and forces which are his by heredity, in order to become a strong, healthy and harmonious human being. It is a fundamental error, to think that the *passive* taking can replace the *active* exercising of our natural functions and faculties.

Of course, there are many other facts which influence man's health and which have to be taken into consideration, such as the pollution of the air, the earth and the water, radioactivity, stresses of all sorts, etc., and means to avoid these noxious influences should be found.

For many decades Chiropractic Colleges have taught postural and spinal hygiene and most Chiropractors do instruct their patients what to do to help avoid recurrence of their troubles arising from the vertebral column but after reading the above it is evident that this is not sufficient.

Today the Chiropractor, if he wants to be a competent counsellor in all questions of health and not only a spinal specialist, must be acquainted with a greater number of causes of disease than was the case some thirty or forty years ago. To be a health counsellor, *he must know and practise himself the laws of health* and be able to explain them to his patients.

Since medicine has failed in this task, this should be a very interesting and very necessary field of study for Chiropractice. "Why aren't we told all that, *about how to stay in good health?*" reflecting people ask when they have become sick through sheer ignorance. Chiropractors should be able to answer these questions of their patients.

The Science of Health is the art of living intelligently. The knowledge and the correct application of the laws of life allow us to live a harmonious, healthy, and happy life. The Science of Health could enable man, instead of degenerating, to advance towards a better and richer life.

A Tribute to B. J. Palmer, D.C., Ph.C. (Scientific developer) and
Mabel Heath Palmer, D.C., M.D. (Co-developer and Anatomist)

"As we pause"

*The full text of the Tribute paid to Dr. B. J. Palmer at the Memorial
Service in Davenport, Iowa, on 31st May, 1961, by Dr. Marcus Bach*

My dear friends, it is quite difficult to speak of B. J. in the past
tense. His presence is so very near to all of us, his influence was so
great and his personality so impressive that the metamorphosis
called death has not yet changed our relationship to him or his
relationship to us. Here was a man who lived not only in time and
space but in spirit, a man whose creativity knew no limiting
dimensions, a man who thought in cosmic terms.

I saw him about four months ago in his Sarasota home. It
seemed to me then that in that frail and failing body was a giant
of indomitable dynamism, the power of some dogged inner will
to live and the secret also of a knowledge that seemed to persuade
him that, despite the indications and reports to the contrary, the
time had not yet come for him to lay aside the physical trappings
that adapt us to this temporal home, the earth.

We cannot yet bring ourselves to speak of him in the past tense
and today, as all of you have gathered in tribute to him, I am sure
that there are many in this vast audience who would be proud to
present a eulogy in his behalf. And because this is true, I do not
want to speak to you unnecessarily, I don't want to speak to
myself, nor do I want to speak to the world, which never understood B. J., anyway. I should like rather to speak to him, so near
does he seem in his presence and his personality.

Because of you, B. J., the world is a better place to live in than
it was before you came. You were a pioneer, and the new frontier
confronting you was a wilderness of sick and dying people, many

of whom had been rejected by medical skills and many had been discouraged by medical science. This was the kind of a frontier into which you came, but it was more than that. It was a frontier also armed to the teeth against any intrusion of its so-called sacred precincts. Anyone who wished to come along with a new idea or a new method stood in danger of being branded a charlatan and a quack, and this is what they often labelled you. But no one knew what God had put into your heart, the *wish* to heal, and no one knew what God had put into your mind and into your hands, the *power* to heal, and no one knew what God had put into your soul, the *truth* about healing. And you took the wish and the power and the truth and you marched across the frontier, stirred and inspired by the secret discovery of your father, D. D., the re-discoverer of Chiropractic, and you marched into a sick and seeking world. You did not march alone; there was faithfully at your right hand, a partner, your wife, Mabel, who by virtue of her own talent became co-founder with you in the school that now bears your name and co-inhabitant in the hearts of those whose lives touched yours.

Because of you, B.J., Chiropractic became a profession and a movement and its exponents in those days were men and women who suffered ridicule and abuse and even imprisonment, so greatly did they admire you and love you, and so determined were they to bring a new technique and a new method into an unbelieving world. It was a new method and a new technique, but it was also as old as time, as old as truth itself, for it was built upon a law, a law that said something like this: God has made man in his own image and God has endowed man with a potential of health, and so long as the channel for the flow of that health can be kept free and open, man cannot be sick, and if man is sick, he can be made well. Jesus called it the God within you; you called it Innate, a word which was used by philosophers of old and which was recognized by your father, D. D., as representing the divine essence of life. You told me once that to you Innate seemed like the God-stuff, the positive centre of life which moved, as you so aptly said, from above down and from the inside out, a phrase that only chiropractors most perfectly understood.

Because of you, B. J., the Palmer School of Chiropractic grew and prospered on Brady Hill. You surrounded yourself with capable men, many of whom are present here today, men who caught your vision and who obeyed and sometimes were in conflict with your will. Students came from all over the world, drawn by your personality. They came not only in search of a career, they came also in search of a philosophy of life, and you gave them both. And many of the students in those days became so infatuated with you that they wanted not only to believe as you believed, and to act as you acted, but they wanted also actually to look the way you looked. This was quite understandable, because you moved through P.S.C. like a major prophet of Chiropractic for more than half a century, a colourful, dedicated, dramatic and sensational figure who never thought in little terms and rarely bothered with little details. You travelled in the days when travel was not easy, and you talked about foreign places and strange sounding people as though they were all part of home town. You brought the culture of the world to Davenport, and you brought the religions of the world to Brady Hill, and you set symbols and artifacts of the world's religions up there long before the most ambitious theologian would ever dare to admit or ever have the vision to see the essential unity of all religions. You built "A Little Bit of Heaven". And you made a prophecy, which is becoming true more rapidly than many people realize, when you said that "All roads that lead to God are good".

B. J., you became a legend in your time, and just about all of the anecdotes and stories told about you are true, and just about everything that is said about your idiosyncrasies are also true. You represented an age and an era, an era and an age that is passing perhaps all too rapidly. This was an era peopled by such personalities as Elbert Hubbard, Calvin Coolidge, Mark Twain, Luther Burbank, and Edwin Markham, all of whom were friends of yours, and you were their friend, and you admired them and they admired you. Something about these men rubbed off on you and I'm sure something of your personality rubbed off on them, and it all was reciprocal and mutual. This was the era of the rugged individualist and you were one of the most rugged, and like the others of your ilk in that particular time, you frowned upon formal academic training and you took a dim

We got to know you as an unusual humanitarian. We knew
you, B. J., as a phenomenal worker, a modern mystic, I would
say, who profounded out a shelf-full of books on his typewriter,
most of them before sunrise. You managed more than a dozen
enterprises, among them the greatest radio and TV station in
Iowa. You will be loved only as a great man can be loved, by
example, and you will be criticized only as a great man can be
criticized, by imitation. In your lifetime, other schools of chiropractic grew up in America and around the world. And something else happened. Many of the forces that fought you have
now begun to examine what you and your father taught and
predicted, and there are some medical circles, as in Germany
particularly, where your technique is already beginning to be
used and appreciated.

There is a strange paradox here, the thousands of chiropractors
who are divided about you are also united because of you. I saw
something of this on the day you died, when, by providential
coincidence, I was addressing a group of chiropractors in the state
of Texas. And I saw these thousand chiropractors, representing
many different schools and schools of thought, I saw them stand
in silent awe when it was announced that you had died, as though
they were trying to comprehend the full impact of your passing.
I heard something else that day, I heard Dave give a talk, and I
realized then that it would have been impossible to have found
a better spokesman for chiropractic than what I heard that day:
remarks that were filled deep with feeling and broad with con-
temporary truth, in which a vision of chiropractic of the future
was projected into time and where it was vowed that in the days
to come the profession would be even greater and more important than it has been in the past. And after that talk, I saw these
thousand chiropractors stand together in agreement in a feeling
that cut across any schismatic lines. Because of you, B. J., we've
gathered here today, in a temple where you so often stood and
with men who knew you well. We are all related to you in
some way, some by blood relationship, some by professional
connection, some by deep bonds of friendship, some by Masonic
ties and other fraternal orders, service club members and friends
from many parts of the world. We are all gathered here, drawn
together most of all I suppose because of love and admiration of a

view of institutionalized religion, believing, and who is to say perhaps not properly, for your particular time, believing that it is possible for man to draw both wisdom and faith from some mysterious cosmic source.

I remember, B. J., how about thirty years ago I sat in a crowded Lyceum tent, unknown and unnoticed, years before I ever spoke from the Lyceum platform. I remember how hot it was that day, but I scarcely noticed the heat, because I had come many miles to hear you speak, and I believe that today I can repeat verbatim many of the things you said. And as I listened to you, I had the feeling that I've often had since that the art of communication is perhaps one of God's greatest endowments to man. I grew to know you through the years and as I grew to know you I grew to love you. And every time one of your new books came out and you sent me one, sincerely and warmly inscribed, I had the feeling that it would be a long time before I or any other man or woman would ever sound or fathom the depth of your thoughts.

You were a cryptic writer of great discernment, and I remember some of the things you said, some humorous, some tremendously profound. You said, I recall, "We look backward upon Jesus with our views, but He looks forward upon us, with his, and what are we going to do about that?" You said once, "We suffer in interpreting Jesus because of the farness, the illusion of the farness of time, and we suffer in our interpretation of Lincoln because of the illusion of the nearness of time." In quoting Napoleon, you said, "Never look upon anything with scepticism or with pre-judgment. Always examine it and find out for yourself what you believe to be truth in it. Remember how Napoleon, after he crossed the Alps in the winter, said to the people, 'Don't praise me for having crossed the Alps, but praise me for not having taken the advice of the fools who said it couldn't be done'." I remember, and many here do, many of the other things you said: "Is life woth living? That depends upon the liver." "It is not man that makes truth great, it is truth that makes man great." "The colour of a man's skin does not in any way detract from his creative contribution, nor does it devaluate his social service." "Make religion your business and make your business your religion."

life so well lived that we will probably go out of this place and want to do a little bit more with the life that is ours.

Because of you, B. J., a great statue will soon be unveiled on Brady Hill, a statue of you, and it will be placed near the statue of your father, D. D. From this vantage point, no less than from the spirit realm, you may watch and participate in spirit in the chiropractic progress of ideas. As generations pass, they will look up and remember you. They will remember, I suppose, most of all, the one word that best describes you, conviction, conviction that you were called into the world by God for a specific purpose, that you had the power and the will to fulfil that purpose, and that every obstacle and opposition were merely tests in the acknowledgement of that purpose. That is the heritage, B. J., that you pass on to us today, and I have no doubt that these moments of tribute and this service today, with the lovely music we have heard and all that we have said and all that we think, will prove to be a time of re-dedication for the members of the profession to which you have so perfectly dedicated the genius of your long and fruitful years.

Marcus Bach, Ph.D.,
Author, Lecturer, Professor of Religion,
State University of Iowa.

DR. BARTLETT JOSHUA PALMER

Developer of Chiropractic

Born 10th September 1881, What Cheer, Iowa.
Died 27th May 1961, Sarasota, Florida (age 79).
Son of Dr. Daniel David Palmer, the Founder of Chiropractic.
Husband of Dr. Mabel H. Palmer, Beloved First Lady of Chiropractic. Father of Dr. Daniel David Palmer, President of the Palmer College of Chiropractic. President of Palmer School of Chiropractic, 1906–1961; the International Chiropractors Association, 1926–1961; a pioneer in radio and television, Central Broadcasting Company, 1933–1961; Tri-City Broadcasting Company, 1935–1961.

B. J.'s keen observation, energy and foresight enabled him to develop chiropractic into a well-defined science.

B. J.'s dynamic personality was behind every phrase of the Chiropractic profession launched in his own colourful and energetic fashion after the death of his father in 1913.

In a lifetime marked by ambition and determination he became, from a modest beginning, the established and acknowledged leader of chiropractice and maintained that position throughout his lifetime. His great ambition was to see the chiropractic principle and practice perpetuate itself in its purity for posterity, unfettered and unshackled by antipodal restrictions, legal or otherwise, so that the sick may have the services of a chiropractor—and the right to a doctor of their own choosing.

He has been eulogized as a genius the world never quite understood; a controversial legendary figure of stature and strength. He overcame obstacles that would have halted many another man. He surmounted long and bitter controversies as he pressed for recognition of chiropractic.

On the occasion of his 75th birthday in 1956, he was presented with the Humanities Award by the North American Association of Chiropractic Schools and Colleges for "adding millions of years to millions of lives".

He wrote an entire library on general and technical aspects of chiropractic and of his world travels, and a book on radio salesmanship.

His monuments also include his unique museum and tropical gardens adjoining his residence. "A little bit o' heaven", opened in 1924, has attracted millions of visitors.

He developed the Palmer School into a world renowned institution with students from each of the United States and from the four corners of the world.

He brought chiropractic into a science with thousands of practitioners and millions of patients the world over.

A man pre-eminent in the history of chiropractic—a many-sided man, a man of numerous qualifications, a canny ability of foresight, unlimited energy, painstaking investigation and research.

DR. B. J. PALMER DIES AT AGE 79

A LEADER PASSES

Following the announcement of Dr. B. J. Palmer's passing by his son, Dr. D. D. Palmer, the editor of the digest of *Chiropractic Economics* asked for the reactions of prominent men in the Chiropractic world. Some of the comments were as follows:

One word describes B. J. Conviction—
Conviction that he was called for a specific purpose, that he was equipped to achieve that purpose and that every obstacle and opposition were merely tests for the strengthening of that purpose. This is what made him great and this is the heritage of greatness he passes on to you and me.

Dr. Marcus Bach

Because of his having lived, millions of years will be added to millions of lives.

Dr. James W. Parker

Only the man has gone—the truths he revealed to the world live on forever.

Dr. Rolla Pennell

Words are inadequate to express my personal feelings of loss. The Chiropractic profession is most fortunate in having Dr. Dave Palmer to carry on the chiropractic torch and the Palmer School, thank God for Dave Palmer. May the profession rally behind him.

George C. Paulk, Jr.

I will always remember B. J. as The Man who made a ladder of his Cross, small in stature, but *great* in courage and perception. To me he was "THE Mighty Atom", my inspiration and guide. I am proud to have been counted amongst his Counsellers and Friends.

Dr. Arthur G. Scofield

I am sure it is not any father image I express when I say that in B. J.'s passing we have lost a father—a loving, scolding, guiding and devoted father who loved me because I loved the things he loved, namely Chiropractic.

Dr. C. S. Cleveland, Sr.

Dr. B. J. Palmer has achieved his place in history through the development of the Science of Chiropractic—writer, teacher, and benefactor of mankind.

Dr. John Q. Thaxton

B. J. Palmer belongs to the ages of men who have made an indelible, beneficial imprint on the history of mankind.

Dr. Bill Harris

He developed the seedling of a great system of healing into a giant power for the benefit of mankind.

Napoleon Hill

We share with all Chiropractic a stunned sorrow as a genius joins the sages.

Dr. Ray LeMond

My grief is that of suffering a deep personal loss, as of that of a relative, even a very close relative; but in a special sense. I do not feel that he will not pass this way again but, rather, that he still lives, here and now, with his eye on all of us.

Dr. C. S. Cleveland, Jr.

As one who has often disagreed with but always loved this monumental man, I say with sorrow and a kind of proud joy what Lincoln's secretary said on the passing of the Great President: "Now he belongs to the ages."

Dr. Marsh Morrison

With his death it seems that man passes and a legend begins. It is difficult to conceive of the Fountain Head without its helmsman. However his spirit will continue to grow and develop through his son as his father's goals were brought to major fruition in his own life. Our profound and sincere condolences go forth to the Palmer family and the entire profession.

Dr. N. Robert Limber

Let us give thanks for a great soul. B. J.'s battle is over, his race is won, his flag waves proudly, his work is well done.

Dr. John Cullum

DR. MABEL H. PALMER (wife of B. J.)

No tribute to B. J. Palmer would be complete unless it included one to his dear wife *Mabel*, and having known her as a personal friend, through student days, graduation, and as a Doctor of Chiropractic, for twenty-six years, up to the time of her passing in 1949, during which years she dedicated her life, side by side, with B. J. Palmer in the development and teaching of Chiropractic at the Palmer College, raising it to its position of pre-eminence in the Chiropractic field.

After graduating from The Rush Medical College, Chicago, Illinois, and founding The Sigma Phi Chi Sorority in 1911 she became as significant a part of the Chiropractic College as her husband B. J.

"Mabel" as she was affectionately known, was credited by all with giving her full strength and courage in the development of the Palmer institution through many trying times.

Possessing a brilliant intellect and a radiant personality, linked with a charming, human, lovable nature as she was held in the highest esteem by all who had the privilege of knowing her.

It was said that her most endearing trait was her kindness and yet without sacrificing this quality, she possessed the glorious mantle of leadership. She had charity and tolerance that bespoke a large soul and the touch of a truly noble woman, genuinely interested in people and their welfare, she was also a diplomat, which quality healed many a professional wound.

She looked for the best in others, and searching for good, found, applauded and portrayed it, giving her a deep faith in humanity.

"Mabel" was revered by thousands of students as a classroom lecturer for over thirty years, teaching Anatomy, sharing with them her philosophy of life, and i n spite of heavy teaching schedules, she found time to write an outstanding book on Anatomy.

DR. DAVID D. PALMER

JOURNEY'S END

Born January 1906. Died May 1978.
President of The Palmer College of Chiropractic since 1961.
Survived by his wife, Dr. Agnes Palmer, and their three
daughters, Bonnie, Jennie, and Vickie.

I was privileged to know Dr. Dave for many years, both as a
friend and, at times, an adviser on professional matters which we
discussed during our many meetings at home and abroad.

The Quad-City Times newspaper carried the following article
on 26th May 1978:

THE LAST PALMER

And now there are none. The name has had such a viable impact
that it is difficult to comprehend a Quad-City Community without
a Palmer.

First, D.D. Palmer, the gruff, bearded, sometimes-eccentric who
discovered chiropractic; then his son, B.J., the wily antagonist who
developed the science and not coincidentally built a broadcasting
and a business empire; and finally the grandson, David D. Palmer,
who finessed it all.

Now, David D. Palmer — the last of the clan — is dead, and he
must be placed in an equal triology with his less retiring forebears.

In all the Palmers, there was something very special that coursed
through their genes; a mix of genius and guts.

But David Palmer had a quality that was lacking in the other
two. Certainly it was compassion — and most especially — patience.
For him, it was not easy to be the son of B.J., the one of 101 talents
and 1001 idiosyncracies, who collected giraffe bones and circus
wagons. David Palmer patiently waited for almost a lifetime to take
over the empire that was so zealously withheld from him by his
father.

And when he did, he sought — and gained — a new respectability
for the science of chiropractic. He created Davenport's first junior
college, without use of a taxpayer's penny; he built an auditorium
where both his basketball team could play and Bob Hope could
preform; he saw the recent dedication of an immense library that
bears his name.

Through his bittersweet life, the past four years have been the
most bitter and frustrating of all. Shackled with the infirmities of a
stroke, he struggled to overcome the handicap, in vain. But his

determination showed best of all the mettle of the man. He refused to give in, and his unbending tenacity became quite clear just a few months ago when he spoke from his wheelchair:

"... I must have the determination to carry on and finish my tasks as a third generation of Palmer should. Though I have had serious setbacks, I see no other avenue of happiness but to get back into the harness, continuing my work with dedication ..."

The community has had but few the likes of David Palmer. He will not easily be forgotten.

In addition, the Vice-President of the Development of the Palmer Chiropractic College, Dr. E.L. Crowder, paid his compliments and respect in the following letter sent to the College Alumni Association members just before the annual Homecoming Seminar:

Dear P.C.C. Alumnus

Every man's life is a plan of God – so it was with Dr. Dave Palmer – and B.J. Palmer – and D.D. Palmer. One hundred and thirty-three years, from 1845, the birth of D.D. to 1978, the death of Dr. Dave, was surely God's calendar of chiropractic design.

Rarely has the world seen and benefitted from such intelligence and positive energy directed to the development and security of a new idea. D.D. designed chiropractic, B.J. developed it, and Dr. Dave, surely in his life and in his death, is giving chiropractic to the world.

Because he was a gentle man and a leader of men, people respected his word. Chiropractic gave him pride; it introduced purpose to his energy and made him pleased with his legacy to mankind.

It may well be he is uncertain we can meaure up to the responsibility and demands of a profession so vital as chiropractic. The Palmer heritage is majestically important to the college and to the profession. We must guard it well lest we also suffer the indignities and lessons of historial precedence. There is no inevitability in history except as men make it. You do not change its course by turning the faces of portraits to the wall. Dr. Dave's life was only the childhood of his immortality.

Homecoming this year will be very special – for him! The David D. Palmer Memorial Homecoming he loved so well.

A Doctor's Viewpoint of Wholefood

Twenty-seven years ago, when I sat in a university lecture room, the Professor of Therapeutics would begin his course of lectures by saying that the active agents, that is those medicines which did any good at all in altering the course of the disease, could almost be counted on the fingers of one hand. Quinine did help malaria, soluble arsenical compounds could bring to a halt the advance of syphilis, liver extract could cure pernicious anaemia—and a few others. But apart from these he would say, "If all the medicines being prescribed in Britain today were thrown into the sea, only the fish would suffer."

Yet even at that time this emphasis on the lack of effective drugs was getting out of date. For in the adjoining wards of Edinburgh Royal Infirmary we were shown patients admitted to hospital suffering from pneumonia who, instead of getting worse and undergoing the harrowing course of this disease, were free from fever in forty-eight hours, sitting up and asking for nourishment.

This was thanks to Messrs. May and Baker's new sulphonamides—the "M and B's"—the magic tablets which were proving to be effective in a number of hitherto untreatable conditions.

And so the new age of medicine was born, the renaissance in doctoring which began in the mid-1930s. A few years later, during the war, penicillin came on the scene and astonished the world with its efficacy. After the war the biochemical revolution quickened its pace.

New broad spectrum antibiotics came fast and in profusion. Streptomycin was found to deter the tubercle bacillus, and at last the conquest of tubercolosis seemed in sight. Cortisone, hypotensives, the tranquillizers, the anticoagulants, poured from the busy laboratories like water from a fountain.

Into the hands of the medical profession had been put sharp, gleaming swords.

The impotence in the face of disease of the doctors of the pre-sulphonamide era, so eloquently expressed by my professor, was a thing of the past and it seems that both doctors and patients have become so dazzled by these outstanding successes in the field of disease treatment that they have been blinded to the simple truth that many of the diseases need never have occurred.

The validity of this simple truth, as I have called it, had been given to the world in 1936 when the late Sir Robert McCarrison delivered his Cantor Lectures before the Society of Arts. He gave the results of his researches into the relationship between food and health, and made a plea for creating a healthy nation on the basis of food which was fresh and whole.

Maybe it was an ironic twist of fate that the new understanding of the *cause* of disease came about the same time as the renaissance in disease *treatment*.

PREVENTION AND TREATMENT

So the medical professions of all advanced countries seem bent on devoting most of their energies to dealing with results, rather than causes.

I think this attitude is well summed up in an opinion expressed in the *B.M.J.* leading article last year..

In an epidemiological survey of dental caries in Ghana, Professor A. B. MacGregor had reported a generally lower incidence of tooth decay than in this country, except in the case of the more wealthy Ghanaians who could afford to buy imported refined flour and sugar. In this group the rate of decay approached that of Britain. As the standard of living in Ghana rises, it was pre-dicted, soon the whole population would be eating, not their own indigenous cereals, but the imported refined carbohydrates. So dental caries in Ghana would become the scourge which it is in Britain. To meet this situation the article suggested the urgent necessity of a crash programme (how planners love crash pro-grammes!) for the training of African dentists. Or, in other words, arrange for a disease to happen and then call for urgent, expensive measures to treat it!

SOMBRE STATISTICS

As a nation, although our mortality statistics have shown steady improvement, we do not appear to get any healthier.

In 1956 the report from the Department of Health for Scotland included this statement, "The hospitals are busier than ever, more outpatients and more patients treated in the wards . . . Morbidity statistics from the Ministry of Pensions and National Insurance show no decline in the incidence of certifiable sickness."

In 1964 the same report stated, "In terms of hospital attendances and demands for hospital treatment it might seem that ill health was increasing . . . There is no simple satisfactory explanation of the fact that better disease control, the saving of lives and improved environment are still accompanied by heavy sickness incidence."

The average number of weeks of sickness benefit for employed men in Great Britain (excluding civil servants) increased from 2·04 weeks in 1959/60 to 2·20 weeks in 1962/63. The increases occurred in all age groups.

In England and Wales the annual rate of discharge from hospital beds for acute illness has been rising from 61 per 1,000 population in 1953 to 70 per 1,000 in 1963.

Some 90,000 schoolchildren in Britain are now leaving school with a full set of dentures.

These are sombre statistics. Seventeen years' experience as a G.P. in a Highland community has not shaken my conviction that improvement will never come about while our people continue their present disastrous dietary habits. Year by year incidents hammer home this truth.

A few years ago I attended a young mother in her first confinement. She was just five feet tall and her father was a farm worker. She had a long, difficult labour ending in operative delivery and a stillborn baby.

Studies in Aberdeen by Professor Sir Dugald Baird have shown that in Social Class 1, that is the professional classes, only 6% of mothers are under 5 ft. 1 in. in height whereas in Social Class V the percentage of small women is 30.

The stillbirth rates in Class V are 50% more than in the professional classes, and the neonatal death rate, that is the death rate of babies in the first month of life, is no less than 100% more.

Here is a classical example of the supreme importance of dietary factors in disease prevention. The small stature of the poorer mothers is due to their inferior diet, their pelvic bones tend to be too small to permit the safe passage of the baby. They are more prone to anaemia, toxaemia and abnormality of all kinds.

I was discussing these things recently in a large hospital with an obstetrician and suggesting that the whole aspect of maternity hospital work would change if only we could upgrade the diet of normal women from Social Class V to that of Social Class I. "Yes," he replied, "and *we* would be out of a job."

EVIDENCE THAT WHOLEFOOD IMPROVES HEALTH

The steepest fall in stillbirths and neonatal death rates occurred during the war. A dramatic improvement which is generally attributed to the war-time food policy—a time when sugar was rationed, the extraction rate of flour was raised and the consumption of fresh milk greatly increased. It cannot have been due to improved maternity service for there was a war-time shortage of doctors and nurses.

But the experience in Holland is even more relevant for those interested in wholefood, because there, although during the German occupation food became scarce, the stillbirth rate fell from 25 per 1,000 births before the war to 19 in 1944. Most of this improvement was due to decrease in toxaemia of pregnancy which is the commonest cause of stillbirth, and the Dutch authorities consider that the improvement was due to the abolition of peacetime overeating. There is other evidence that a high intake of refined foods such as sugar and refined flour is the main cause of pregnancy toxaemia.

Dr. E. H. Hipsley reported some time ago in the *B.M.J.* the results of surveys of pregnancy toxaemia in Fiji. Among the Eijian women studied the incidence of toxaemia in the years of study was zero, whereas in the Indian community living in Fiji it was relatively high. The Fijian diet consists of fresh vegetables, fruits and small quantities of meat, fish and crabs, the bulk of the Indian diet is refined flour and rice.

This experience agrees exactly with a delightful essay written by Dr. Mary Jackson on her work in Northern Alberta among the Metis Indians. She went there in 1930 and for the first twelve years never saw a case of pregnancy toxaemia.

But during the war the Mackenzie Highway to the northern oilfields and uranium mines was driven through this territory. The Indians were given highly paid jobs and access to imported food.

Instead of fresh meat, fresh fruit, beans, eggs and the flesh of fish or birds, they began eating white bread, sugary processed breakfast foods, puddings, sweet biscuits, candy and chocolate. For the first time cases of pregnancy toxaemia began to appear. To quote Dr. Jackson, "So a rising standard of living, and a considerable measure of social security have been accompanied by an increase in the incidence of dental caries and a falling standard of health in pregnant and old people."

How often, as the cause of a disease is finally explained after patient, complex research, the case for dietary reform is strengthened! Here again I quote from personal experience.

In 1959 I attended a tinker woman in her second pregnancy. The tinkers have a social class zero of their own. Their menfolk are seldom in constant employment and so depend on public assistance; they live a hand-to-mouth existence on the cheapest food. Thorough ante-natal care in this case was impossible as the woman wouldn't come to the surgery and was constantly shifting her tent. After having her baby in our hospital, she developed a swinging fever, and severe gastro-intestinal symptoms. I thought she had gastro-enteritis or dysentery and sent her to the isolation hospital. There examination of her blood showed that she was suffering from macrocytic or megaloblastic anaemia of pregnancy. In 1961 another tinker, who early in her pregnancy was found to be gravely anaemic, proved to be suffering from the same complaint. Both these women improved rapidly on being given tablets of folic acid. This is a vitamin which, as its name suggests, is found in green leaves of vegetables and to a lesser extent in wheaten flour; it is easily destroyed by cooking. Attention to its action was first published by Dr. Lucy Wills in 1938 when she was studying this megaloblastic anaemia in Bombay among people whose diet consisted mainly of white bread and polished rice. The diet of my tinker patients is probably not much better.

Folic acid is essential for the normal production in bone marrow of the blood's red cells. Without it cell production becomes abnormal and the circulating red cells progressively fewer.

But more recently it has been shown that folic acid deficiency is also associated with some cases of premature separation of the placenta and deformities of the foetus. The former carries high mortality for the baby and grave dangers for the mother.

This vitamin is related to nucleic acid of cell nuclei and is essential for growing tissue, hence the extra need for it and its tremendous importance throughout pregnancy. Studies have shown that deficiency precedes manifest anaemia. A recent survey by bone marrow puncture of a random group of pregnant women showed that no less than 25% of subjects showed signs of megaloblastic or abnormal cell development. Deficiency of this vitamin in pregnancy is thus fairly widespread especially among Social Class V.

So advice to pregnant women to eat whole wheat bread and one raw salad dish becomes not the ravings of a crank, but sound dietary advice based on most recent research. The enterprising drug firms have been quick to develop a pill containing both folic acid and iron and these are now being routinely prescribed in many ante-natal clinics. But I have read of no authorities questioning the habit of putting essential food factors in a pill, which should come from our plates.

CORONARY ARTERY DISEASE

I wish to turn now to one of the most terrible epidemics of modern times, coronary artery disease. (There is no general agreement among medical authorities about the cause of the tremendous increase in the last three decades, of disability and death due to this disease.)

One fact is undisputed—primitive races, having as yet no contact with "civilized" foods, show an almost complete absence of this heart disease below sixty years of age; but when these same people have access to "civilized" food they start getting the disease. An interesting example of this was recently published in *The Lancet*, giving information about the changed dietary habits in Israel of settlers from the Yemen. Newcomers from the Yemen had been shown to suffer much less from coronary heart disease, high blood pressure and diabetes, than did their fellow Yemenites who had been settled in Israel for more than twenty-five years.

Doctors Cohen, Baily and Poznanski, who did this work, suggested that the chief cause for this deteriorating health might be the increased consumption in Israel of sugar. In the Yemen no refined sugar was taken by the families studied, whereas when they settled in Israel it formed about 20% of their carbohydrate. Otherwise their diets were broadly similar.

My own feeling is that fats do not play such an important part and that, when the final truth is exposed, this disease will be yet another example of—to quote Cleave—"saccharin disease"—a condition due to diets over-heavy with refined carbohydrates.

If dietary factors cause degeneration of arterial walls it might be expected that other tissues in the same patient would also be affected by degenerative processes.

DIET, STRESS AND HEREDITY

Occasionally studies of individual cases for which the G.P. is so well placed may be as revealing as the wider surveys of the epidemiologist.

I followed the cases of two men with serious degeneration of the intervertebral discs of their spines and both later developed fatal coronary artery blockage. I believe that the causes of these two quite separate conditions is the same dietary inadequacy. Degeneration of intervertebral discs seems to be another condition on the increase and it is my opinion that the main cause is inadequate or unbalanced intake of minerals and possibly lack of protein or vitamin factors.

Another thing I have noticed is the frequency with which, on examining many of the people who succumb to coronary thrombosis while on holiday in our practice area, the tell-tale scar of gastrectomy—that is the operation to "cure" duodenal ulcer—is found in the same patients. This is an impression, with no figures to back it up, but Fry, in his practice near London, has given statistical evidence to suggest that there is an association between peptic ulcer and coronary thrombosis.

"But wait," the protagonists of psycho-somatic medicine will say at this point, "the association, if it exists, between the two diseases is because both were caused by the same emotional stress."

My reply would be that the body and mind were built to withstand both physical and mental stress. I sometimes wonder if some people in this Britain of today couldn't do with a bit more stress! I think of the parable of the two houses, one built on sand, the other on rock. When the storms of stress blow hard the in-adequately fed organism, nourished on the deprived foodstuffs of today, will wear out or collapse. An adequately nourished organism will stand.

Probably hereditary factors determine which system or organ will break down first when the individual is exposed to adverse dietary factors.

Two bachelor brothers lived on a hill farm. They were not over-intelligent and the squalor of their kitchen was terrible to see. Their feeding arrangements consisted in getting from the weekly van what could satisfy hunger with the minimum of trouble, and white bread with jam, tea, tinned milk and tinned meat seemed to be the main items on the menu. Two years ago one brother developed a painful leg. He was found to have profound anaemia and massive haemorrhages typical of scurvy. But the other brother was unaffected, possibly his metabolism was better adapted to utilizing the slender supplies of available Vitamin C.

These two brothers might be termed modern-day primitives, their small farm from which they seldom strayed is surrounded by luxurious growth of green things, mostly nettles and other weeds. What a sad reflection that they had lost even the instinctive sense to cultivate a few potatoes or turnips.

Not far away by the road, an old lady almost ninety sits by her fire and speaks, as is usual in the aged, of the days gone by and deplores—again as old people do—present-day customs. We can ignore her opinions, if we like, as being the ramblings of senes-cence, but her account of the nutrition of her childhood is interesting. "We had plenty of everything on our farm," she has said to me. "We had cows and sheep and hens. We made lovely cheeses and lots of fresh butter." I know the old lady's farm. The pastures have gone out of cultivation, and some of them have been blotted out by the Forestry Commission's economic, dark green conifers. The farm house is the weekend cottage of a professor of economics from a distant university.

The picture of the decay of the Highlands' vigorous rural economy and its inhabitants is a depressing indictment of our modern age.

THE REMEDY IS TOO SIMPLE

The other day I came across a remarkable echo of "The weakness of the remedy lies in its simplicity". James Lind, the Portsmouth Naval Surgeon who had suggested that scurvy among sailors could be prevented by a ration of lemon juice, wrote, "Some persons cannot be brought to believe that a disease so fatal can be prevented by such easy means. They would have more faith in an elaborate composition dignified with the title of an anti-scorbatic golden elixir or the like."

Although we have seen in recent decades a tremendous expansion of human knowledge of material things, I doubt if we have matched our increase in knowledge with a deepening of our wisdom.

Over huge tracts of our lovely country we have created an appalling urban environment which rots our lungs and starves our souls. In Scotland we have created wilderness where once was cultivation, and ruins where once was community.

A Prelude to the talk

"The Power Within"

Arthur G. Scofield, D.C., F.P.A.C.

About ten years ago, Dr. R. W. Johnston wrote as follows:

"Most of us accept as fact the existence of a Creator, a power much greater than man, who in his wisdom created the Universe and all that it contains. Some call this power God, some The Almighty, some the Creator, many refer to it as just Nature. Be that as it may, there is an acknowledgement by all classes, including the Scientist and Atheists, of all races and creeds of a supreme driving power of such vast organized control, that man as such, cannot duplicate, and, call it what you will, it is still the same."

The re-discoverer and developer of the Chiropractic Profession called this power "Universal Intelligence" and in all the books written by B. J. Palmer, in order to differentiate between the three sources of bodily control—the outer force or power is referred to as Universal Intelligence; the continuation of this within the body is referred to as *Innate*, meaning inborn; while its adaptive use within the body by association with education is termed the Educated Mind.

Now Universal Intelligence, when creating this Universe, laid down certain fundamental laws which govern our very existence. We often think of certain laws (Newton's law of gravity, for example) as being man made. This, of course, is not true, for it is one of *nature's laws* which existed since the beginning of time. If it were not for this law we would not cling to the surface of the earth but would be flung into space as the earth spins on its axis.

Because of the Laws of the Universe we have such things as day and night, rain and shine, winter and summer, autumn and spring. Our existence on this earth depends on these changes, and they come about naturally and automatically without our help. Just imagine how terrible it would be if it were daylight all the time, winter all the time, or if the rains never came.

The balance in Nature is too comprehensive and far reaching to have just happened. It must have been planned. Snow falls on the mountains in the winter. With the advent of spring the snow melts into water which runs down the mountainside, becoming part of the great rivers which flow across the wide plains to the ocean.

In their course they water the land, provide us with water for many things, thereby contributing to the well-being of all.

Every creature, regardless of size, has its place in the scheme of things. Large animals live on smaller animals, and small animals live on insects and plant life. If it were not so the world would be over-run with many types of animals or plant life, and there would not be a balance in nature.

Many times man executes huge engineering feats which seem wonderful and necessary at the moment, but if, as a result of these, the balance or plan of nature is interfered with, disastrous results will take place, perhaps years later. (We have had an example in Wales where, through the spewing of vast heaps of slag taken from the mines and dumped without order or planning in the lovely countryside of Wales, has resulted in the premature death of scores of innocent children). The area involvement is no doubt small when compared to the hundreds and thousands of miles that can be affected by disturbing nature without adequate planning.

In the United States, for example, man has built on the great Colorado River many dams to provide hydro-electric power as well as to irrigate many arid acres of land. Now this river flows over many miles of the American continent, finally emptying itself into the Gulf of California.

Before these dams were built tons of silt were carried down the course of the river, deposited at its mouth, thereby creating a natural sea wall which prevented sea water from entering Death and Imperial Valleys in California, both of which are below sea level. Now a good proportion of this silt is collecting behind the dams built, and only a very little is finding its way to the mouth of the river.

The result of this is that the natural sea wall is not being maintained, and if Death and Imperial Valleys are to continue to support the people they now do, and remain free of sea water, man is going to have to build a sea wall to take the place of the natural one. In this instance man, due to lack of foresight, has upset another of nature's laws of balance, and as a result, will be forced to undertake another huge project involving millions of dollars, or suffer the severe flooding of thousands of square miles of fertile land involving thousands of people.

Returning to *our* Science, you will remember the reference to the continuance of a Universal Power or Intelligence coming from without, entering and controlling our life through the second interpretation of internal power, which we will refer to as Innate, or the Inborn power. This power built our human living bodies, she knew how to build them, she drew the blueprints, organized every organ, assembled them, started and keeps them running. She put life into each and all of them, knew just how to economically put together all parts, and how to keep life existing in them. Innate directs, regulates, governs and controls all functions, in all bodies, all the time. She knows when something is wrong, where, how much, what needs re-building, and how to do the same. She is the one eternal, internal, staple, permanent factor that is a fixed and reliable entity, does not fluctuate, or violate its own self-made laws.

The same internal natural intelligence which knows when to sneeze, blow your nose, blink your eyes, how to heal a cut, or mend a fractured bone, raise a blister when the skin is burned, grows hair, nails, and tells you when you are thirsty, hungry, or sleepy; all this and more is the same capable inner "voice of power" to get any sick organ well.

"The Power Within"

"God breathed into man the breath of life"

How often have we heard that expression during our lifetime? I remember it so well when first taken to a church service. I tried to visualize the act, got confused and gave up trying, but often it came back to me and eventually I filed it in a wee corner of my brain, along with my attempts to visualize the creation of the earth, the stars, the planets and just where did all that material come from that made up those celestial bodies? It is still there tucked away in its little niche, and I realize that one could spend a lifetime in contemplation and still get nowhere, so I divide my time, one in the world of phantasy, and the other in as practical a manner as possible, which enables me to use and apply what known facts exist and interpret the force that produced them.

In an earlier chapter I mentioned the interpretation B. J. Palmer used in describing "Life without" as a universal intelligence, "life within" as innate intelligence, and man's use of this power as educated intelligence, and that the uninterrupted expression of the power within through "innate" produced health, therefore B. J. Palmer appropriately considered that God breathed into man the "breath of life" and, he added, left within a manager to regulate bodily functions including the reproduction of cells.

There is a power within you which you recognize as the ability to move-see-hear-speak-breathe, what is this power? Who can answer? We call that power "Innate Intelligence", you look around and recognize some power that governs and controls the universe and all things in it, you may call it nature, you may call it an act of God, but it is still a vital force.

Within you is a grain of the universal power, if there was not, you would cease to move, see, hear, breathe, feel, or exist as a human being.

As long as that power within you has control of your body a

state of health exists, should something interfere with your
normal control of that internal power, then you would cease to
enjoy your birthright of "Health".

Science has taught us to recognize when dis-ease exists and,
notwithstanding the fact that so-called diseases in specific areas
are named as such; cardiac disease, kidney disease, stomach
disease or, more specifically, terms such as valvular heart disease,
ulcerated stomach disease, nephritis, describing a form of kidney
disease, often the reason for the dis-ease is the inability of your
internal power, "Innate Intelligence" to properly regulate body
functions.

In Chiropractice we maintain that your "innate" controls all
bodily functions through the nervous system, if some factor causes
a disturbance in the nerves that would interfere with thought
transmission from the brain or source of such an impulse to the
nerve endings, be it the organ, tissue and/or periphery, then at
the end of that nerve you begin to feel the state of disease, health
being a state maintained through innate having 100% control
of your life through the nerves of your physical body.

Chiropractice is a method used to release interference to nerve
supply so that the "power within" can heal you. Our instruments
tell us when trouble in the nerves has developed, our spinographs
give detailed information of the state existing at the point of
interference, and our adjustments to the spinal vertebra correct
the causes when they exist, releasing pressure from nerve roots,
thereby enabling them to function normally.

The Doctor of Chiropractic does everything possible to help
innate heal your body by removing obstruction causing interference with the distribution of nerve impulses, but healing is a
process afforded you by your Creator and is above and beyond
the control of man.

No doctor can heal, nor can anyone else produce healing for
you, but when the correct adjustments are made, innate (the
power within) goes to work and you feel the results when *dis*-
ease turns to ease. Which reminds me of the patient that told me,
"I don't think you are doing me much good, but these pills
seem to be working at last." Little did that patient realize that
the removal of nerve interference had given the body a tolerance
to the drug content, and had also kicked the chemical balance

over to its favour, and the patient credits the drug and not his own body ability with his recovery.

Within the human mind and body we have two distinctly different personalities, "*Innate* and *educated*" intelligence, these live in two distinctly phased sections of the brain. "Innate" is on the job twenty-four hours a day, every second from birth to death and during "waking hours" it permits certain portions of external body to be under the direction of "educated intelligence", just so long as what that educated personality does is not too destructive, but during "sleeping hours" educated personality is dormant, not present, and innate is in full control of all parts, and if during waking hours educated mind or intelligence drives the body to function in a way that would be detrimental to continuity of life's expression, then innate would induce "sleep" which is a voluntary withdrawal of innate from superficial portions of "educated body" thus forcing it into a non-conscious state for the time being. "Fainting" is also a voluntary withdrawal of innate from superficial or educated body.

At all times, under all circumstances, Innate is in full and complete control of the body, knowing whether or not to induce "sleep" depending upon the necessities of that body for rest and recuperation.

Universal Intelligence. In B. J. Palmer's book, *Law of Life*, he states: "In our humble opinion Webster's definition of universal intelligence limits it to being within the narrow confines of what man thinks of as 'education' which is more or less the passing of viewpoints from one person to another, or from reading books which express opinions of other people." Our concept of universal intelligence goes beyond any understanding of human beings.

Any attempt to put into language an interpretation of that overall guiding intelligence fails. It comes, it is, it does, without language, what it alone sees fit to do.

Universal Intelligence supplies the power whereby innate intelligence within the mother builds the unborn child. In due time it is ushered into the world connected to the mother by the umbilical cord, and until the cord is severed the child is wholly dependent upon the mother, but once the cord is cut and the newborn baby gives that first squeal or cry it is an independent unit or being.

What was it, that "something", entering that body in one second, which caused it to live? Can you who read, think, see and hear a child come to life, do better? The education of the father or mother did not bring this transformation about.

As parents you do not beg, borrow, steal or buy "it"; neither do you see It enter the baby body, It comes, It permeates matter, It lives, what was it? Who knows? We acknowledge it, we recognize its presence as SOURCE, what more can we do?

When innate intelligence (the power within) enters, the full, free flow, mental impulse is turned on, the chemical laboratories within the body begin to function, many substantial mechanical parts begin taking on definite motions, after which the former inanimate matter becomes animate, something which is not a material thing, but an abstract something has taken its place and is directing yet another human being. How futile are words, and how humble is man, when he tries to describe this metamorphosis in attempting to explain this phenomenon.

The innate of mother, building a new child, is another job in a woman's life; giving it birth is a process of necessity which even she does not comprehend; getting its breath of life is a common occurrence in the routines, these are beyond man's pale of understanding, and what he cannot understand is a miracle; or Feat of Nature.

Life however with its supply of universal intelligence, expressed and controlled by the innate intelligence within the child, progresses through childhood, adolescence, and adult life, and during its progress through these stages of growth he gets knocked down, set up, strained, undernourished at times, and overfed at other times.

Within man's body the chemical laboratory works continuously to maintain a normal balance between insufficiency and excess, it repairs a break in the tissue, knits torn muscles, mends that fracture, and removes scar tissue that protects injured places whilst the healing process goes on, and this little understood power within us spends its life preserving, repairing and maintaining our spirit through many a hard test of time.

The Power Within knows just when to stop the baby's growth at the end of its childhood, just how tall and wide and deep its body must develop to be properly balanced, just when to stop multiplying cells around a deep cut, when to create a callous to protect skin and muscles from friction, just how much lime, calcium, potash salts, etc., are required to mend a broken bone, and when to remove the protective bursa around that fracture. This power within will serve you throughout your natural life, providing it can reach the organs or parts by means of uninterrupted nerve distribution.

However, there sometimes exists a blockage along the pathway of the nerves that supply the energy and movement to these vital regions, due to a partial misalignment of the vertebrae surrounding the body's major lifelines emanating from the spinal cord and there follows a reduction of nerve energy to organs and parts often accompanied by changes in glandular and chemical balance. It is then that the doctor of chiropractice is able to assist nature by adjusting vertebral misplacements thereby removing pressure interference where nerve roots are affected, and where sometimes increasing pressure threatens direct effect to spinal cord and possibly life itself, and by so doing the 'lengthening shadow' is changed to the lengthening light.

Doctors of Chiropractice are therefore making a valuable contribution to longevity increasing the numbers of those reaching the eighties and nineties, and I think within the lifetime of the children born this year it will be possible for many more to reach the century mark.

If chiropractice succeeds in wiping out acute and chronic disease, then humans should and will live, actively, usefully, and cheerfully with full mental powers to the day they die. B. J. Palmer once said a human being ought to live until he wears out, not rusts out, he ought to die as the light of a candle goes out, burning with a bright flame to the end of the wick, then a short spluttering, dimness, a final splutter and darkness.

There should be no ancients in the chimney corner, a man ought to possess his full powers to the day he dies, his light as bright as the brightness of the candle before that final splutter.

It is a beautiful idea, that of a poet and a dreamer, but it *is* logical, why should one man be on the shelf for years before he dies, while others in these days of knowledge and great civilization seem to even increase their mental powers until the end?

"The only death ought to be the sudden death of ripe old age."

Glossary of Chiropractic Terminology

ADJUSTMENT:
The art or procedure of adjusting spinal bones by hand to release pressures on the nervous system.

ANALYSIS:
The term used to denote the findings by a chiropractor after checking the spine for any nerve interference or pressures. A name is not given to the symptoms caused by the nerve pressure because his corrective work is based on correcting the cause rather than treating the symptoms: effect.

ATLAS:
The first or topmost vertebra of the spine.

AXIS:
The second vertebra of the spine.

ATLAS/AXIS REGION:
Pertaining to the region of the spine occupied by the first and second vertebrae.

ATLANTO-AXIAL:
Pertaining to the region of the first and second vertebrae.

CHIROPRACTICE:
A system of adjusting by hand the vertebrae of the spinal column; the term was derived from two Greek words (Cheir) hand, (Praktos) done by, literally means done by hand.

CERVICAL:
Neck region, the first seven vertebrae of the spine.

CORRECTION:
A term used to denote an adjustment of a spinal misalignment or subluxation.

DIS-EASE (Disease):
Lack of ease, lack of co-ordination of any body tissues or organ with the total organism due to nerve interference.

DORSAL:
Mid-back, next twelve vertebrae below the cervical region.

FORAMEN MAGNUM:
Great opening in the occipital bone through which the brain and spinal cord are connected.

INNATE
  INTELLIGENCE: The resident inborn intelligence within each individual unit maintaining and co-ordinating body function by way of the nervous system. Sometimes referred to as sub-conscious mind or Nature.

INTERVERTEBRAL
  FORAMEN: Passage for spinal nerves and vessels between adjacent vertebra.

LUMBAR: Low back region, next five vertebrae below the dorsal area.

MENTAL IMPULSE: Impulses created in the brain and directed over the nervous system causing tissue cell function.

NEUROCALOGRAPH: An automatic thermo-coupling graph recording instrument which records minute heat variations on corresponding sides of the spinal column.

NERVE PRESSURE: See Nerve Interference.

NERVE INTERFERENCE: Pressures on the nervous system particularly in the region of the intervertebral foramen. Pressure on nerves causes loss of normal function which may result in pain, paralysis, or any symptoms which, if given a name, could be called Sciatica, Neuralgia, etc.

NEUROCALOMETER: An instrument which detects minute heat variations on corresponding sides of the spinal column, invented by D. Evans, and introduced to the profession by B. J. Palmer.

ORTHOPAEDIC
  SURGERY: Manipulation as practised by members of the medical profession.

OSTEOPATHY: A system of body mechanics founded by Andrew Taylor Still in 1894 based on the premise that faulty structure or disturbed structural homeostasis can affect physiological functioning detrimentally.

READING: A recorded result of instrument check for evidence of nerve pressure or interference.

RETRACING: A condition sometimes experienced following spinal adjustments whereby the patient experiences similar symptoms to those present when dis-ease is developing. Usually of short duration.

SPINAL BALANCE TECHNIQUE: A system of Chiropractice once taught at the Universal College, Pittsburg.

SPINOGRAPHY: A specific technique development for taking x-rays of the spine to ensure the maximum contrast pictures.

SACRUM AND COCCYX: Spinal segments below the lumbar area forming the base of the spine.

VERTEBRAL SUBLUXATION: A term used to denote a condition in which vertebrae (the bones of the spinal column) are out of position to such an extent that a pressure, or interference, is produced at the nerve roots, with subsequent inflammation producing discomfort or dis-ease.

X-RAY(s):   A discovery by Röntgen the same year (1895) that D. D. Palmer re-discovered Chiropractice.